DISCARD

# ENCYCLOPEDIA OF
# FAMILY HEALTH

—— THIRD EDITION ——

# ENCYCLOPEDIA OF
# FAMILY HEALTH

## THIRD EDITION

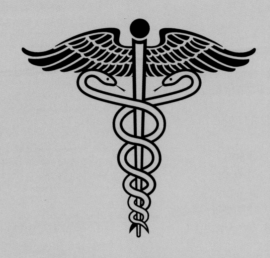

CONSULTANTS

David B. Jacoby, M.D.
Johns Hopkins School of Medicine

Robert M. Youngson, M.D.
Royal Society of Medicine

# VOLUME 15

# SPASTIC COLON — SYRINGING

MARSHALL CAVENDISH
New York • London • Singapore

## MEDICAL CONSULTANTS

Second Edition
David B. Jacoby, M.D.
Johns Hopkins School of Medicine
Associate Professor of Pulmonary and Critical
 Care Medicine

Third Edition
Robert M. Youngson, M.D.
Fellow of the Royal Society of Medicine
Officer of the Order of St John of Jerusalem
Diploma in Tropical Medicine and Hygiene
Fellow of the Royal College of Ophthalmologists

## CONTRIBUTORS TO THIRD EDITION

David Arnot
Deborah Evans
Leon Gray
Joanna Griffin
Tim Harris
John Jackson

Tom Jackson
Nathan Lepora
Fiona Plowman
Alison Tarrant
Aruna Vasudevan

**Marshall Cavendish**
99 White Plains Road
Tarrytown, NY 10591-9001

www.marshallcavendish.com

© 2005, 1998, 1991 Marshall Cavendish Corporation

Library of Congress Cataloging-in-Publication Data

Encyclopedia of family health / David B. Jacoby, Robert M. Youngson.--
3rd ed.
        p. cm.
Includes bibliographical references and index.
 ISBN 0-7614-7486-2 (set)
 ISBN 0-7614-7501-X (vol 15)
1. Medicine, Popular--Encyclopedias. 2. Health--Encylopedias. 1. Jacoby, David
B. II. Youngson, R. M. III. Marshall Cavendish Corporation. IV. Title
RC81.A2E5 2004
610'.3--dc22                                          2003065554

Printed in China
08 07 06 05 04 5 4 3 2 1

**Marshall Cavendish**

Editor: Joyce Tavolacci
Editorial Director: Paul Bernabeo
Production Manager: Alan Tsai

**The Brown Reference Group**

Project Editor: Anne Hildyard
Editors: Jane Lanigan, Sally McFall
Designers: Jeni Child, Reg Cox, Karen Frazer
Picture Researcher: Clare Newman
Indexer: Kay Ollerenshaw
Illustrations: Samantha J. Elmhurst
Managing Editor: Tim Cooke
Art Director: Dave Goodman

# CONTENTS

Spastic colon 2022
Specimens 2024
Speculum 2027
Speech 2028
Speech therapy 2032
Sperm 2034
Sphygmomanometer 2036
Spina bifida 2037
Spinal cord 2040
Spleen 2044
Splinters 2047
Splints 2048
Sports injury 2050
Sports medicine 2052
Sprains 2056
Stammering and
    stuttering 2058
Staphylococcus 2062
Starch 2063
Stem cell 2065
Stenosis 2067
Sterilization 2068
Steroids 2072
Stethoscope 2074
Stiffness 2076
Stillbirth 2080
Stimulants 2083
Stitch 2086
Stomach 2088
Stomach pump 2091
Strangulation 2094
Streptococcus 2097
Stress 2098
Stress management 2103
Stretch marks 2105
Stroke 2107
Sty 2112
Subconscious 2114

Sudden infant death
    syndrome (SIDS) 2116
Suffocation 2118
Sugars 2120
Suicide 2122
Sunburn 2126
Sunstroke 2130
Suppositories 2132
Surgery 2134
Surrogacy 2141
Sutures 2144
Swellings 2145
Symptoms 2149
Syphilis 2153
Syringing 2156
Index 2158

KEY TO COLOR CODING OF ARTICLES

HUMAN BODY

DISEASES AND OTHER DISORDERS

TREATMENTS AND CURES

PREVENTION AND DIAGNOSIS OF DISEASE

HUMAN BEHAVIOR

# Spastic colon

**Spastic colon is a distressing condition. It is a variant of irritable bowel syndrome, and is classified as a functional (nonorganic) disorder, but so far there has been little progress in discovering its cause.**

"Spastic colon," a term not universally approved by doctors, but widely used, is now generally recognized as one of the varieties of the functional bowel disease known as irritable bowel syndrome (see Irritable Bowel Syndrome). Doctors have found difficulty in categorizing functional bowel disease because the symptoms suffered, although genuine and distressing to the patient, are often difficult to explain in terms of conventional pathology and physiology. In 1990, a working group was set up at the 13th International Congress of Gastroenterology in

## Questions and Answers

**My husband died of colonic cancer and my 22-year-old daughter suffers badly from spastic colon. She is terrified that she, too, will develop cancer. Is this likely? And if not, how can I reassure her?**

Cancer of the colon is a common disease but is very rare in people in their early twenties. The average age at diagnosis is between 60 and 65. Spastic colon, on the other hand, is common in young adults. In addition, the symptoms of the two conditions are entirely different and there is no evidence that spastic colon leads to cancer. Perhaps this will help reassure your daughter.

**My friend, who is 31, has been diagnosed with spastic colon. I believe that the condition is the same as irritable bowel syndrome, but she disagrees. She says that IBS is all in the mind but that spastic colon is a genuine disease. Which of us is right?**

It is true that spastic colon and irritable bowel syndrome have much in common and that many doctors make no distinction between them. But the experts now consider that spastic colon is one of the variants of irritable bowel syndrome. Most important of all, however, is the fact that they are both real, distressing conditions; they are not imaginary.

**Has spastic colon got anything to do with cerebral palsy?**

Nothing whatever. Cerebral palsy, also called spastic paralysis, is present from birth and affects the voluntary muscles. Spastic colon is an adult disorder and affects the involuntary smooth muscles in the walls of the bowel. The two conditions could hardly be more different. The only thing they have in common is muscle spasm.

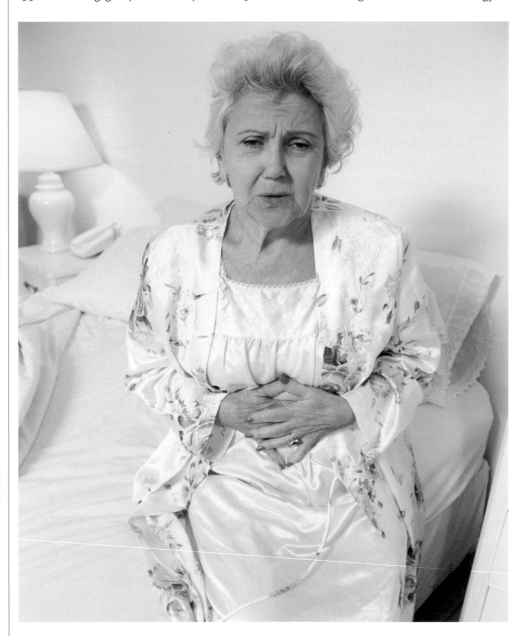

▲ *Uncomfortable abdominal pain is characteristic of spastic colon and irritable bowel syndrome. Antispasmodic drugs will help relax the contractions of the digestive tract.*

Rome, and its recommendations, known as the Rome criteria, are widely accepted. One of the categories in the Rome criteria, based primarily on symptoms, is spastic colon. This condition affects women much more often than men.

## Symptoms

The main symptom is pain. This is often sudden, sharp, severe, and piercing, and is located in the lower abdomen just above the pubis. Often, the pain is of short duration and may be associated with the passage of loose stools. There may be distension of the abdomen and a sense, after defecating, that the act has been incomplete so that the affected person feels the need to defecate again. Mucus is commonly present in the stools. Frequently, the abdominal pain will be relieved by defecating.

Diarrhea is not, however, a principal symptom of spastic colon and although it is quite common for sufferers to feel the need to go frequently to the toilet, constipation is a common feature. Spastic colon may be very persistent and chronic and can be a severely debilitating condition (see Diarrhea).

## Causes of spasm

Spasm, which causes the digestive tract to contract suddenly, involuntarily, and abnormally, results in pain and distress for the person affected. Most people have experienced muscle spasm in the form of painful cramps. Common cramps are spasms of the voluntary skeletal muscles. In the case of spastic colon, however, the muscles concerned are smooth, circularly-placed muscles in the wall of the intestine that are not under voluntary control but contract because of the action of the nerves of the autonomic nervous system. The symptoms of spastic colon strongly suggest that the normal mechanisms of bowel peristalsis are disordered. Peristalsis, which is produced by organized contraction of the walls of the intestine, is necessary so that the contents of the bowel can be moved along. This is achieved by a process in which, about three times a minute and at many points along the intestine, a short segment of bowel constricts while the adjacent segment, on the side of the constriction nearer the anal end, relaxes. The effect is to force the food contents along. Peristalsis operates throughout the whole length of the gastrointestinal tract and involves the gullet and stomach as well as the small intestine and colon.

Any disturbance of the peristaltic mechanism—as when, for instance, two closely adjacent segments tighten strongly so that a length of bowel balloons between them—will produce sharp pain. It is known to medical science that the intestine is completely insensitive to touch and even to cutting or burning, but it has numerous sensory nerve endings that respond sharply to stretching. The difficulty is to discover what it is that brings about the irregularities or abnormalities in the mechanisms of contractility and peristalsis.

It is because there is a disorder of bowel function, rather than an actual structural disease that could be revealed by biopsy, that this condition is called a "functional disorder." The term should not be interpreted, as it often is, as meaning that this is an imaginary complaint. Some research suggests the possibility that at least some cases of spastic colon, especially in black people, may be due to lactose intolerance. Lactose (milk sugar) requires the enzyme lactase for its digestion, and in its absence undigested sugar ferments in the colon, causing diarrhea and distention.

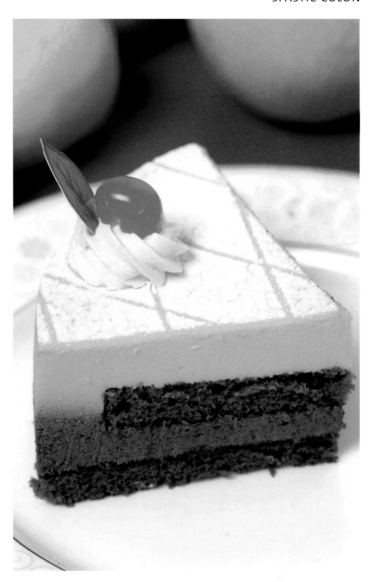

▲ *People who suffer from spastic colon sometimes find that certain foods exacerbate the problem. Generally, fatty foods, such as this slice of cake, should be avoided.*

## Treatment

Although the cause of the disorder remains uncertain, that is no reason why it should not be treated. Although doctors always attempt to discover the cause of a disorder and then try to remove that cause, they recognize that there are some conditions in which it is legitimate to treat symptoms without knowing their exact cause. Spastic colon is such a condition (see Symptoms).

There are several drugs in the category known as smooth muscle relaxants or antispasmodics, and these can be effective in relieving the symptoms of spastic colon. They include dicyclomine (Antispas), glycopyrrolate (Robinul), hyoscyamine (Anaspaz), propantheline (Pro-Banthine), and mebeverine hydrochloride (Colofac). These drugs work in different ways, and trials may be necessary to find out which is best for any particular patient. If diarrhea is a main feature of the condition it can be controlled by small doses of loperamide (brand name, Imodium) taken as needed.

> *See also:* Colon and colitis; Diet

# Specimens

**What would be found in a urine sample taken during pregnancy?**

During pregnancy, the placenta produces human chorionic gonadotropin (HCG), which is detectable from about six weeks. It is produced in increasing amounts during pregnancy and is excreted in the urine. Its presence in the urine almost always means that the patient is pregnant.

**Are specimens of skin tissue ever taken to diagnose skin disease?**

Yes. This may be done to diagnose fungal infections and skin cancer, which can often be completely cured, either by removing the abnormal skin and a thin rim of normal skin around it, or by radiotherapy. A skin sample may also be taken to rule out skin cancer, which mimics many other conditions, and to identify the exact disease, because this will affect treatment. Taking a specimen of skin is usually a simple procedure which can be done under local anesthesia.

**Why does every patient in a hospital have a blood test?**

Sometimes blood tests are done to look for a specific disease such as anemia during pregnancy. Often, blood is taken as part of a screening procedure, and is subjected to tests that are most likely to help diagnosis. Every patient has a urine test for sugar, blood, and protein, which may show unsuspected diabetes or kidney disease.

**Can an unborn baby be tested?**

Yes. The amniotic fluid can be tested to reveal deformities or blood group incompatibilities between mother and baby. The baby sheds cells, which can be cultured and tested.

**Taking a specimen from someone is usually a simple, painless procedure, and the information it provides can be invaluable in the diagnosis and treatment of disease.**

Most people have had a blood or urine test at some time. These are the most common of a wide range of samples which may be taken from the body's tissues or fluids to assist in diagnosing a disease. A huge number of specimens are sent daily to pathology laboratories where detailed analyses are carried out. The physician's skill in piecing together his or her patient's symptoms is supported by extensive laboratory data (see Diagnosis; Pathology).

Specimens can be taken from all body fluids and tissues. Blood and urine are the most common because they are easy to obtain, relatively cheap to test, and very useful in diagnosis. For just a routine examination blood and urine tests can reveal serious diseases, such as anemia, leukemia, and diabetes. A range of more detailed tests of blood and urine are routinely used in clinical medicine (see Laboratory Tests).

## Blood tests

In addition to the assessment of the number and appearance of the red blood cells and of their hemoglobin content, blood is commonly examined for the presence of some of the many specific enzymes and antibodies it may contain (see Blood). When heart muscle is damaged in a heart attack, certain enzymes are released into the blood from the affected cells. A measurement of the levels of such enzymes can give an accurate assessment of the amount of heart muscle affected and hence of the severity of the heart attack and the probable outcome (see Heart Attack). The process is similar when the liver is damaged by infection or poisoning.

Blood antibody levels are among the most important of the many tests that can be performed on blood specimens. Modern techniques of identification and the level of antibodies present allow very precise diagnosis of previous infection. Many hundreds of different conditions can be identified in this way.

For most blood tests, a specimen of blood may be taken from a vein in the arm using a syringe and fine needle. In some cases it is sufficient to prick a finger and obtain a drop of blood. There

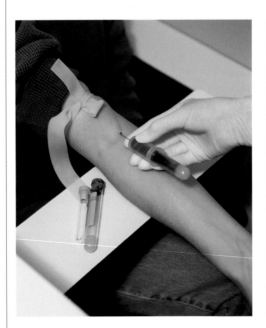

▲ *Vein punctures are used to remove blood to be used for laboratory tests.*

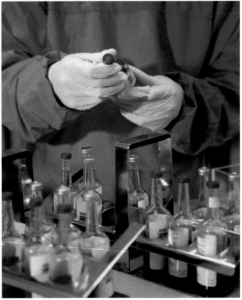

▲ *A technician checks the labels on sample bottles in a laboratory.*

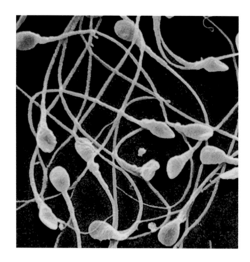

▲ *In cases of infertility, a sperm sample is examined for abnormalities.*

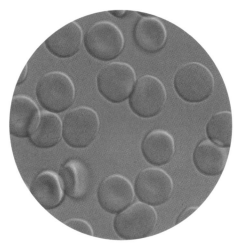

▲ *Blood analysis is a routine but invaluable aid in diagnosis.*

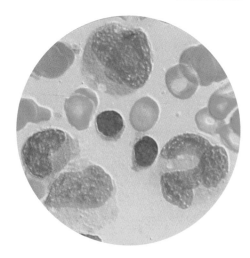

▲ *A bone marrow smear can indicate leukemia and rare types of anemia.*

are conditions, however, in which it is essential that a specimen should be taken from the bloodstream in the heart or in the large vessels running to or from the lungs. If this is the case, a fine sterile tube called a catheter is passed through a vein or an artery and threaded along to the required point. Analysis of blood gases (oxygen and carbon dioxide) from these sites can provide vital information about the condition of the lungs and the heart.

### Urine and stool tests

Urine tests can detect many diseases, including diabetes, which is indicated when a urine specimen is found to contain sugar. Although many of the urine tests indicate disease of the kidneys, one or more of a wide range of abnormal constituents may be present, which can indicate disease of other organs or parts of the body.

Samples of stool (see Feces) are commonly taken to help in the diagnosis of a wide range of intestinal disorders. Stool samples can be tested by sensitive chemical analysis for blood that is present in such small quantities that it is not apparent to the naked eye. It is known as occult blood, and its presence can be highly important in various conditions that include cancer of the large intestine and amebic dysentery.

Chemical analysis of the stools is commonly performed to assess the fat content when it is suspected that dietary fat is not being absorbed efficiently enough. Characteristic fatty stools result when a patient is suffering from malabsorption. Failure of protein digestion can also be detected by analysis of stools.

Another test that is carried out on stool specimens is a search for the eggs of intestinal worms. A small quantity of the specimen is shaken up in salt water. A drop of the suspension is placed on a microscope slide and covered with a cover glass, which is a layer of very thin glass. The eggs of parasites differ in subtle details from each other. This characteristic appearance can be detected by a pathologist or technical expert so that a precise identification of the type of parasite can be made (see Parasites).

### Sputum tests

In cases of chest infection, sputum can be cultured to identify the infecting organisms present, and their sensitivity to a selection of antibiotics can be determined. In suspected tuberculosis, sputum is stained and examined under a microscope, and other tests can be done to identify the causal organism. In lung cancer, sputum will often contain cast-off cancer cells that can be identified by an experienced pathologist. If meningitis is suspected, the cerebrospinal fluid that circulates around the brain is examined, and fluid from a swollen joint can be analyzed to determine the cause. Sputum can provide evidence of infection or cancer.

### Biopsies

It is possible to take small samples of tissue from organs (see Biopsy) without using open surgery. Flexible tubes, or endoscopes, can be

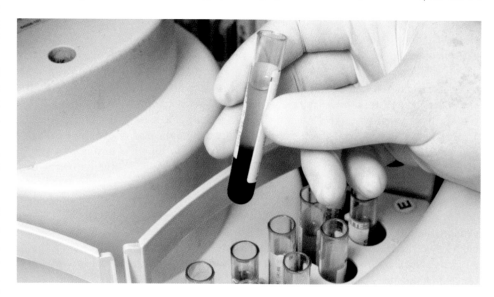

▲ *Many types of chemical and hematological blood tests can be carried out on an autoanalyzer, which, as its name implies, automatically analyzes samples.*

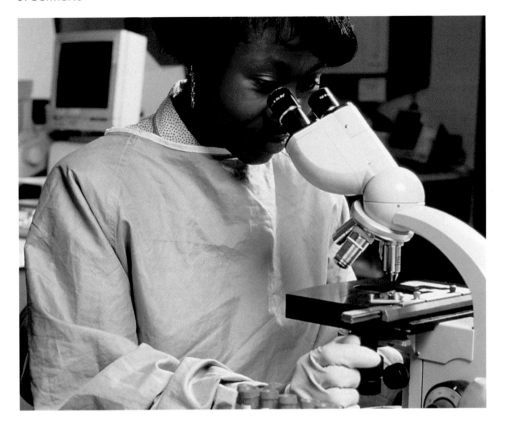

▲ A laboratory technician can learn a great deal from an examination of blood samples for the presence of enzymes and antibodies.

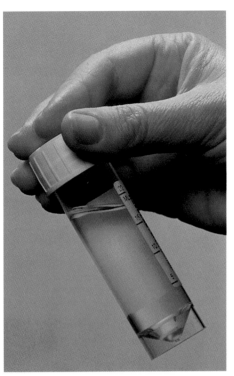

▲ Biochemical analysis of urine is used in the diagnosis of conditions such as diabetes, and for the detection of illicit drugs.

inserted into the stomach and along the rectum and colon. Small pieces of tissue may then be removed for examination under a microscope. Similarly, pieces of the liver, kidneys, and bone marrow can be obtained using fine, rigid tubes or special probes and needles. Even such vital organs as the heart and brain can have tiny biopsies removed and examined. This method of sampling tissue is not without risk, but most of these procedures have become routine and the hazards are minimal (see Endoscopy). Biopsies are the most reliable way of making a diagnosis and will usually be required if a serious condition, such as cancer, is a possibility (see Cancer). Histopathology is the subdivision of general pathology concerned with the microscopic examination of tissue specimens obtained by biopsy. After the tissue is processed, extremely thin slices are cut using a micrometer; they are then placed on glass slides, stained, and examined. Histopathologists are experienced in recognizing subtle changes that occur in cells and tissues as a result of disease and can determine with a high degree of reliability the presence of many different diseases.

### Why a specimen is taken

The main reason for taking a specimen is to confirm a diagnosis. A doctor will seldom feel confident about making a diagnosis without supportive evidence from an examination of blood, urine, or a tissue biopsy. Blood and urine tests are particularly useful in monitoring the progress and treatment of disease. An example is of some types of cancer that secrete substances into the blood. As the cancer responds to treatment these substances will disappear, so in such cases regular blood tests are an accurate means of charting the course of a disease. Finally, specimens may be taken as part of a screening program to detect latent disease. No disease is suspected in any individual, but if enough people are examined, some cases will be found. The aim must also be to detect the condition at an early enough stage so that effective treatment can be given.

The best example of this is a cervical smear test, which is intended to detect early cancer of the cervix (see Pap Smear). Cells from the cervix are removed and spread on a glass slide for examination under a microscope. Many cases of cancer that are discovered in this way are still at an early stage, and treatment usually effects a complete cure.

### Processing specimens

Often the most simple test gives the most information; more may be learned from examining a blood film than from any other laboratory test, yet the specimen is easily obtained and prepared. Routine testing of urine is also simple and straightforward, but unexpected diseases may be diagnosed in this way. It is vital to ensure that specimens do not get mixed up, so each laboratory in the pathology department takes the utmost precautions to guard against this possibility. All labeling is checked at every stage and errors hardly ever occur. Routine analysis is carried out by a specially trained laboratory staff. The results of the tests are sent directly to a patient's doctor. Any abnormal results are usually shown to a relevant pathologist, who will advise clinicians about the significance of abnormal results. The best procedure to follow can then be discussed. The pathologist reports on all tissue samples.

*See also:* **Bacteria; Lumbar puncture; Symptoms**

# Speculum

**A doctor uses a speculum to examine various passages in the body or to assist in administering medication. A speculum can help a doctor to make a diagnosis without causing the patient too much discomfort.**

I would like advice about contraception from a family planning clinic before I have sexual intercourse. Will I need a pelvic examination, and if so, will it be painful?

Pelvic and vaginal speculum examinations are performed at family planning clinics to establish that the reproductive organs are healthy. It is very unlikely that a virgin will have any abnormality of the cervix. Because of this, and because an internal examination may be uncomfortable if you have an intact hymen, most gynecologists would delay the internal examination until you have experienced intercourse.

I had a miscarriage just after an internal examination, during which a speculum was used. I am pregnant again and am worried that the same thing might happen again. Is an examination really necessary?

There is no evidence that a gentle internal examination will cause a miscarriage, although your anxiety is understandable. You should explain this to your obstetrician. Much useful information is gained by a pelvic examination early in pregnancy and a speculum is used to check for infection in the vagina and to examine the cervix. Your obstetrician may, however, be prepared to avoid doing this if he or she feels that it will cause you great anxiety.

My gynecologist says he has difficulty inserting a speculum into my vagina. Why is this?

If you are tense, the muscles surrounding the vagina go into spasm and narrow the vagina instead of allowing it to expand as it is when relaxed. Perhaps you could learn to relax more when being examined by concentrating on deep breathing exercises.

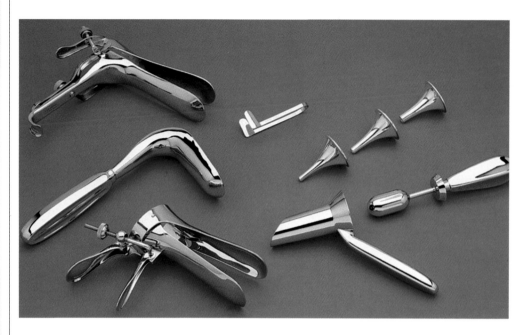

▲ *The three vaginal specula often used are Grave's, Sim's, and Cusco's, shown top to bottom on the left of the picture. Those on the right are for nose, ears, and rectum.*

To make an accurate diagnosis of some conditions it is necessary for the doctor to look into various passages of the body—for example, the ear, nostrils, vagina, or rectum. An instrument that is designed to help a doctor to do this is called a speculum (plural, specula). Depending on what a speculum is used for, it will vary in shape and size. Most specula are made of highly polished metal which will reflect light well. Disposable plastic specula are also available.

To use a speculum, it is gently inserted into the passage to be examined. The doctor initially separates the walls at the entrance of the body passage with his or her fingers to facilitate the entry of the speculum.

## The vaginal speculum

The most commonly used vaginal speculum is the duckbill-shaped Cusco's speculum. When the blades are separated they divide and completely cover the opposing sides of the vaginal walls, so that the cervix can be seen. It is possible to take swabs of vaginal and cervical secretions to check for genital infection. It is also possible to check that the thread of an intrauterine contraceptive device is in place and to take Pap tests.

The cervix can be examined in the same way (see Pap Smear). The Sim's speculum is another commonly used vaginal speculum. It enables a doctor to examine the vaginal walls for prolapse, ulcers, or atrophic (thinned) mucous membranes. The speculum is used to depress the front or back vaginal walls and reflect light onto the opposite wall, enabling that wall to be examined easily.

A nasal speculum is used to help the doctor look for foreign bodies, polyps, or very fragile blood vessels, which may cause the patient to have frequent nosebleeds.

A speculum that is frequently used is one for examining the eardrum and the external canal of the ear.

> **See also:** Cervix and cervical smears; Contraception; Vagina

# Speech

Anyone who has ever lost his or her voice for some reason will know how extremely frustrating it can be not to be able to communicate. Speech, one of humans' most essential and flexible abilities, is indeed a precious faculty.

Speech is one of the most complex and delicate operations that the body is asked to undertake. Ultimately all speech, talking, and comprehension are controlled and coordinated by the brain, and it is in the cerebral cortex that there are areas called the speech centers where words are deciphered and signals and instructions are sent out to the many muscles in the face, throat, and mouth that are involved in producing speech (see Brain; Muscles; Throat). All this complex control is something that people are born with the ability to do, but the actual way people speak and the sounds they make are learned from their parents and the people around them as they grow up.

**My son does not speak very clearly, and we can't even make out what he is saying at times. Should we be worried or is he just going through a lazy phase?**

If you think your son has a speech problem, take him to your doctor. The doctor may be unable to find out the exact nature of the problem but will be able to refer him to a specialist for further tests and diagnosis if necessary. It is unlikely that his poor speech is caused by laziness, particularly if the defect is bad enough to make him hard to understand. A child may grow out of a genuine speech problem but as time goes on the problem could get worse, so it is essential that he sees a doctor.

**My son is two years old and has not made any attempts at speech. All my friends' children of a similar age started speaking some time ago; should I be concerned?**

It is not unusual for children, especially boys, not to speak until around the age of two. After this time they usually make excellent progress and catch up quickly. As a precaution, take your son to your doctor, who will be able to assess him and, if need be, send him to a speech therapist for further examinations. If there is a genuine reason for his slow speech development, the cause can be any number of things, from the purely physical (an abnormality of the voice box) to a deep-seated psychological problem. Whatever the cause, early diagnosis is vital, because if there is a defect, the earlier it is corrected the better the outcome. If the delay in developing language is marked, there can be an associated problem in learning the rules of syntax and grammar. Dyslexia or word blindness, for instance, can be associated with problems of speech development; some people believe that dyslexia is more common than was previously thought.

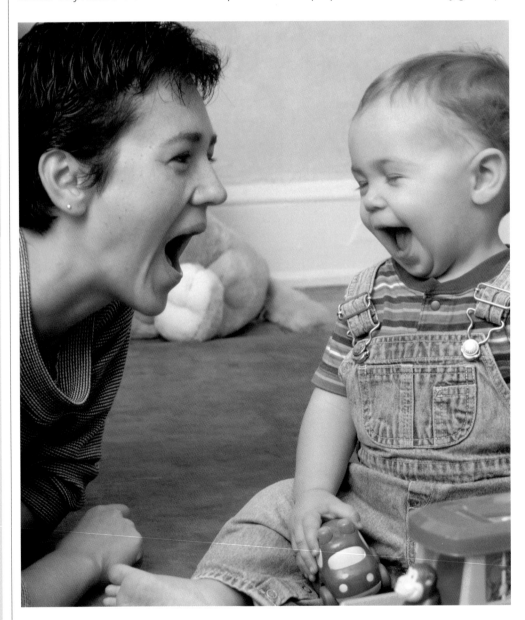

▲ *This 16-month-old child is learning to talk by imitating the physical movements of his mother's mouth and the sounds that come from it.*

## Thinking and speaking

The cerebral cortex of the brain is divided into left and right sections called hemispheres. Speech and its associated functions are usually concentrated in one hemisphere; in a right-handed person this is usually in the left hemisphere, and in a left-handed person it is usually in the right hemisphere. This area of the brain is divided into the motor speech center, which controls the muscles of the mouth and throat; and the sensory speech center, which interprets the incoming sound signals coming along the nerve from the ears. Also nearby are the parts of the brain that coordinate hearing (by which people comprehend what others are saying), vision (by which they decipher the written word), and the complex hand movements used in writing, playing an instrument, and so on.

Conversation is a very complicated procedure, and the first thing that happens when a person hears another person speaking is that the hearing centers, in the cerebral cortex, recognize the jumble of incoming auditory signals from the ears (see Hearing). The sensory speech center decodes the words so that the other parts of the brain involved in the process can then recognize the words and formulate an answer. Once a reply has been thought up, the motor speech center and another part of the brain, called the brain stem, come into operation. The brain stem controls both the intercostal muscles, between the ribs, which inflate the lungs; and the abdominal muscles, which determine the pressure of the incoming and outgoing air. As air is expelled from the lungs, the motor speech area signals the vocal cords simultaneously to move into the stream of air in the throat, causing the cords to vibrate and produce a simple sound. This is called phonation.

The amount of pressure applied to the lungs during exhalation governs the speed with which the air passes over the vocal cords, and the faster the air, the louder the sound produced. During whispering the vocal cords are set wide apart so that they do not actually vibrate as the air passes between them, they merely act as friction surfaces. For the most part, however, the shaping of words is performed by movements of the lips, tongue, and soft palate—controlled by the cortex.

## Producing words

To turn the simple sounds produced by the vocal cords into intelligible words, the lips,

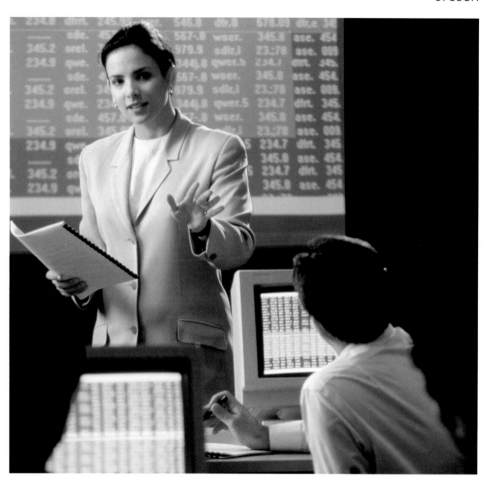

▲ *In job training sessions, the instructor must be articulate, and be able to speak clearly and directly to trainees.*

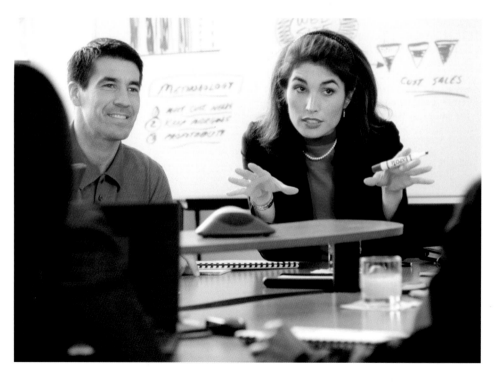

▲ *This woman is chairing a business meeting. Her ability to structure her speech and be articulate and concise with words will affect her success in the business world.*

## Questions and Answers

**My husband suffered a stroke some time ago which left him partially paralyzed. This also made him lose his powers of speech. What can be done to overcome his problem?**

Loss of the power of speech (aphasia) may be due to the inability to understand words or the inability to express them, or both. Some degree of spontaneous recovery is common, but if this does not occur within a matter of weeks it is unlikely that speech therapy will help. It should always be tried, however. The method that might be used to retrain your husband would involve laboriously repeating words and phrases and the rules of grammar, just as a child would when initially learning the language. This would be supervised by a speech therapist.

**I have been told that the only way to cure my child's speech problem is to send him to a special school. Is this really necessary?**

Treatment of some speech defects can be a long and subtle process and is often most effective under confined and controlled conditions available at a special school. Treatment at a special school could last about three years, after which time the child may be able to return to a regular school. The length of time that the treatment lasts varies, however, depending on the cause of the child's problem.

**What can be done for someone with a cleft palate, and is treatment effective?**

A cleft palate is a gap or a cleft in the roof of the mouth or upper jaw. This condition is usually treated in babies immediately, or soon, after birth. The fissure is closed by surgery. If a cleft palate is not treated until after the person begins speaking, speech therapy is used to clear up any language defects that may have developed. Today, a cleft palate does not have any real effect on the way a person speaks, since the surgery available mends the damage completely.

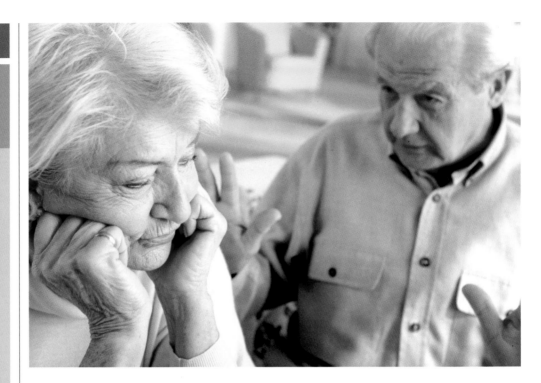

▲ *Arguments are another area in which the ability to present one's thoughts and feelings reasonably and precisely can help other people to understand the problems at hand.*

the tongue, the soft palate, and the chambers, which give resonance to the voice, all play a part. The resonating chambers include the whole mouth chamber, the nose, the pharynx (the part of the throat between the mouth and the esophagus), and to a lesser degree the chest cavity (see Chest; Nose; Pharynx). The control of these structures is achieved by many muscles that work very closely together and at incredible speed. Put simply, speech is made up of vowels and consonants; vowels are all phonated sounds.

The resonant qualities of the various chambers of the mouth and respiratory system provide people with the individuality of their voices. For instance, the so-called nasal sounds like "m," "n," and "ng" depend for their correct vocalization on free resonance in the nose; if a person pinches his or her nose when speaking, the comic effect shows how the airspace of the nose gives the speech roundness and clarity. Everyone has a differently shaped nose, chest, and mouth; therefore different people have different-sounding voices.

The skull also resonates when people speak, and people hear part of what other people say transmitted through the bones of the skull, as well as what is picked up by the ears. This not only provides a person with vital feedback about what he or she is saying, but also explains why the voice sounds so strange when played back through a tape recorder—the sounds a person then hears being only those transmitted through air.

### Learning to speak

The rate at which children acquire the power of speech varies from one individual to another, but the same landmarks in speech development normally occur in all growing children. For up to three or four months after birth, most of the sounds a baby makes are those used in crying. After this the baby starts to make speechlike sounds when gurgling and babbling. These noises are thought to be common to babies of all different nationalities, and are even found in babies who are deaf (see Deafness). This has led many people to conclude that the capability for language is inherent in all people.

At around four months of age the baby starts to coo and chuckle, and toward 10 months sounds heard around the infant may be repeated. From 10 to 12 months the first audible words are usually produced. These words are often nouns naming the things that the infant sees around him or her or mean that the baby is asking for something with one word.

From 12 to 18 months the child jabbers tunefully while at play and uses between six and 20 recognizable words; the child also understands many more words. From the age of two the

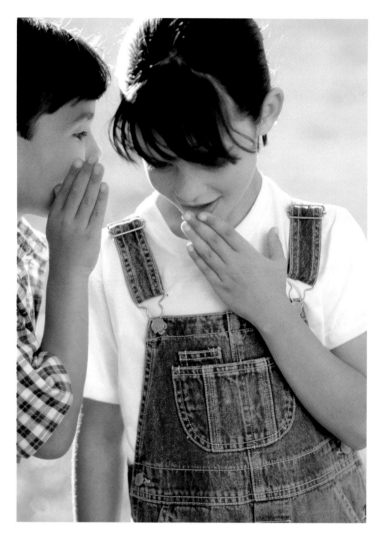

▲ *As children develop their speech as they grow older, they are increasingly able to control their speech volumes as appropriate, from shouting to whispering.*

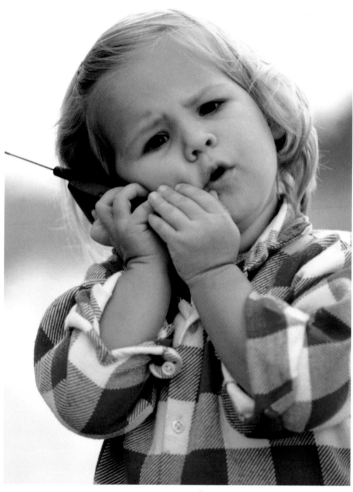

▲ *Toddlers will sometimes practice their speech by pretending to talk to other people on the telephone.*

structuring of language begins and more than two or so words are strung together at one time. Also, the child starts to pick up the idiomatic meaning of groups of words. From three to five years, sentences become longer and convey a more exact meaning, and basic grammar is gradually mastered. From school age, development of speech becomes more structured as vocabulary and grammar are learned in a more systematic manner.

One great asset that people possess is inquisitiveness, and this is nowhere more evident than in a child who is learning new words and phrases every day.

## Speech defects

Because of the great complexity of the whole speech process, involving as it does many areas of the brain, the control of breathing, and all the many muscles that manipulate the sound-producing and sound-modifying apparatus, speech problems can be very complicated.

The disorders can be divided into several types: problems of the voice (disorders of the larynx and its parts); problems of voice development; problems caused by damage to the various speech areas of the brain; abnormalities of the mouth; and problems brought on by or associated with deafness. Basically, anything that

gets in the way of the ability either to formulate speech (in the brain), communicate the commands to the bodily parts (along the nerve network), or execute the commands (in the muscles) can cause some kind of speech disorder.

Some disorders caused by problems with the nervous system are called dysarthria (see Nervous System). In this category are diseases such as cerebral palsy, shaking palsy, and chorea (see Cerebral Palsy). Deafness can cause mutism because a deaf child will not be able to pick up the language being spoken around him. If the patient is deaf at birth, concentrated speech therapy must be undertaken using visual means to stimulate the correct vocalization of words.

These are some of the areas where there are problems with speech, and treatment depends on the actual cause of the disturbance. The determination of the cause can involve consultation with neurologists, psychologists, or any of the other specialists involved with the speech-producing mechanisms (see Neurology and Neurosurgery). Any eventual treatment may involve doctors and therapists from many specialties.

*See also:* **Aphasia; Child development; Dyslexia; Larynx and laryngitis; Mouth; Mutism; Palate; Speech therapy; Tongue; Vocal cords**

# Speech therapy

For stroke victims or children with a speech impediment, speech therapy plays a vital role in helping people to communicate clearly and thus live as normal and happy a life as possible.

## Questions and Answers

**My child has a stutter that seems to be getting worse. What can be done to stop it?**

A speech therapist will be able to decide whether your child is just going through a phase of poor speech, often called disfluency, or whether the stuttering is more than a phase. The therapist will also decide if it is appropriate to intervene with treatment. If so, he or she will teach your child how to speak more easily and assist you, through parent counseling, on how to help your child at home between visits to the therapist. Most cases of stuttering clear up spontaneously.

**What training do speech therapists have, and where do they practice?**

Speech therapists have at least a master's degree. Subjects covered include child development, phonetics, linguistics, psychology, anatomy and physiology, neurology, and speech pathology. They work in schools, hospitals, rehabilitation centers, speech and hearing centers, and speech clinics.

**My three-year-old son can hear but does not speak. Should I take him to see a speech therapist?**

Children, especially boys, often do not speak until quite late. If you are worried, go to your doctor, who may refer you to a speech therapist who is trained to correct language difficulties including delayed speech and development.

**My father has Parkinson's disease. His speech is faint and hard to understand. Where can I get help?**

At the speech therapy department of your local hospital. A speech therapist will be able to treat your father's speech by training him to speak more slowly and distinctly.

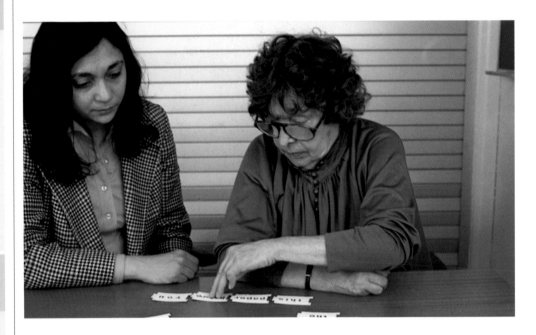

▲ *This stroke victim is at an advanced stage of recovery. She is being asked to rearrange word cards into relatively complicated sentences. Often stroke victims have to learn language anew.*

Many people confuse speech therapy with elocution or teaching people to pronounce English clearly, but a speech therapist is not someone who changes accents or dialects. He or she helps children and adults who have speech or language difficulties that make it hard for them to understand or be understood by other people (see Stammering and Stuttering). A speech therapist is responsible for assessment, diagnosis, and treatment of any speech or language difficulty, usually after the patient has been referred by a doctor.

### Speech difficulty

The main areas in which people need speech therapy are difficulty in understanding speech or language; difficulty in articulation (pronunciation of sounds); and difficulty in expressing ideas through spoken, written, or sign language. Some of these problems may be the result of a stroke or an accident (see Stroke).

Causes of speech or language difficulty in children include delayed development or disorder of articulation (pronunciation of sounds), delayed or disordered development of language, physical or intellectual impairments, autism, cleft palate, deafness, voice disorder, and stammering. Adults can suffer from speech or language problems, caused by stroke, Parkinson's disease, multiple sclerosis, or cancer of the larynx (see Multiple Sclerosis; Parkinson's Disease).

Difficulties in understanding and expression of speech and language vary enormously. In children, problems usually result from damage to the brain, hearing, or speaking apparatus from birth, or delayed and sometimes abnormal development in childhood. Adults usually lose the ability to speak as a result of brain damage, or damage to the nerves that supply the speech muscles, or the deterioration of the muscles of speech through disease. In some cases of cancer of the larynx the whole voice box is removed, and the patient has to learn to speak using the esophagus (see Esophagus).

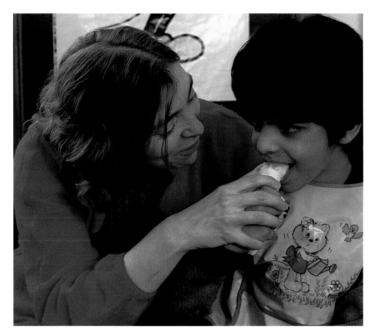

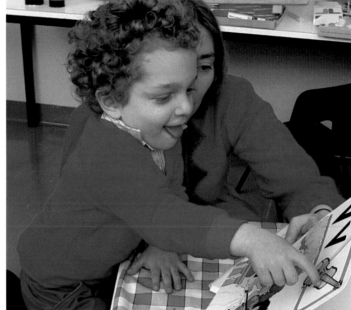

*▲ ► Speech therapy applies many techniques in the effort to restore lost speech or aid late development. Children who have been in accidents often have to be helped to try even the most basic of speech-related exercises. Having to stretch the mouth to accommodate a banana will exercise the muscles, and blowing out candles will help the child to control breathing and form the lips into one of the basic shapes used in the production of speech. A child with delayed speech development could be asked to point at pictures of items mentioned by the therapist. In all cases the therapist aims to make the session fun.*

### Therapy for children

Unless the child's difficulty is purely in speaking, or the speech problems are very severe, the first area of treatment is language comprehension. In young children between the ages of three and six years this is usually done through play. The parents also take a major role in continuing therapy in between sessions with the therapist. Typically, language is taught by play, for example with a doll's house, with items of furniture, and miniature people. In short and simple language, the child is asked to select items—this teaches nouns. The child is then asked to do things with them—this teaches verbs.

When children have difficulty in articulating, it is usually because they either do not know how to make particular sounds, or they do not recognize that certain sounds are different from other similar ones. The ability to express all sounds is not usually complete until the age of six or seven, so a speech therapist would not treat a four-year-old who had difficulty with only "s" or "r" sounds because these are difficult sounds to speak. In therapy, a child is first shown how to make the sound. He or she then says the sound only before going on to practice it as the first sound in short words. The child then says the sound at the end of words and finally in the middle of words before trying to use it in continuous speech.

### Therapy for adults

When speech or language is lost through brain damage as a result of stroke, the patient often recovers some or all of his or her speech

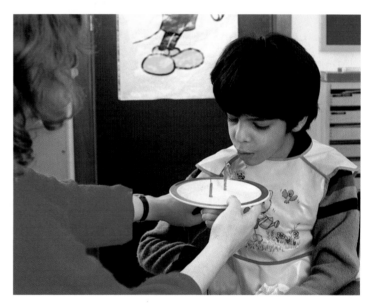

spontaneously, usually between six months and two years after the stroke. The speech therapist's role is to guide and stimulate recovery with speech and language exercises. The exercises include pointing to pictures by name and reconstructing complex, abstract sentences in which written words have been jumbled.

The extent of recovery depends on the extent of brain damage (see Brain Damage and Disease). Some patients never recover speech and language. If that is the case, other forms of communication are taught, which may include simple gestures or sign language, or the patients' pointing at pictures of what they need.

Slurred articulation, called dysarthria, is often caused by a stroke or multiple sclerosis, and occurs because the tongue cannot move rapidly enough from one sound to another. Patients are taught to slow down their speech, allowing time to make the sounds accurately. Tongue and lip exercises are practiced in order to strengthen the muscles of speech.

---

*See also:* **Speech; Vocal cords**

# Sperm

**Is it true that a man can become infertile by wearing tight trousers?**

Yes, to a degree. Tight trousers and nylon underwear may increase the temperature inside the testicles to a point where sperm production simply stops, but this is only a temporary condition.

**At what age does a young man start to produce sperm, and for how long does this continue?**

Sperm are first produced at puberty, at about age 12, and production continues throughout the life of a healthy male. Even a man of 90 is able to father a child.

**If sperm are of poor quality, could the child be unhealthy or damaged?**

About 20 percent of sperm in the typical ejaculate are abnormal, but such sperm are normally unable to fertilize an egg. If fertilization occurs, the result is often spontaneous abortion—nature's way of coping. Substances such as lead have now been found to cause fetal abnormality where damaged sperm were previously suspected.

**A test showed that I have a low sperm count. What does this mean and will it improve?**

The sperm count is the number of sperm in each milliliter of seminal fluid. Between 2 and 5 milliliters are normally ejaculated at each orgasm. Sperm counts may vary according to the body temperature when the sperm is formed or the frequency of intercourse, but if your sperm count is consistently below 20 million per milliliter and there is no treatable cause, it is unlikely to improve. However, you may still be able to father a child; it may be possible to artificially inseminate using your sperm. A subfertility clinic can advise on this.

**The human male is an amazingly prolific producer of sperm: up to 350 million are released in one ejaculation. However, only one sperm may complete the journey to the female's egg and achieve fertilization.**

"Sperm" is the name given to the male reproductive cells—the spermatozoa. It is also commonly used as another word for seminal fluid, but in this article it is used only to refer to both the single spermatozoon and the plural spermatozoa.

The sperm's only purpose is to achieve fertilization by union with the female cell, the ovum. Each sperm is about 0.002 inch (0.05 mm) in length and shaped like a tadpole. It has three main sections: a head, a midsection, and a tail. The front of the head—the acrosome—contains special enzymes

## HOW SPERM MATURE

▼ *From puberty, sperm are constantly produced in the seminiferous tubules. To become sperm, the basic sperm cells go through three stages of cell division (bottom) before passing through the tubules and into the epididymis, where they are stored (below left). A mature normal sperm has a head, midsection, and tail (below right).*

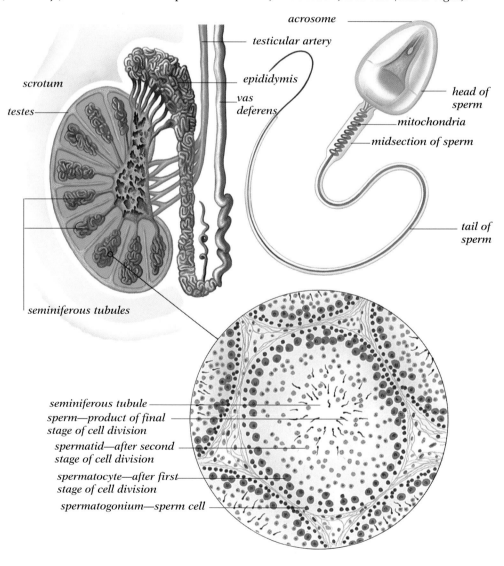

that enable the sperm to penetrate into the ovum and achieve fertilization (see Enzymes). The midsection contains structures called mitochondria. These structures hold the vital source of energy needed by the sperm to fuel it on its journey to the ovum.

The tail's only function is to propel the sperm, which it does by moving in a whiplike fashion, generating a speed of about 0.12 to 0.14 inch (3 to 3.5 mm) per minute.

Sperm are made up of a number of essential chemicals and genetic material. These are the chromosomes that carry the genetic blueprint of the father and determine the paternally inherited characteristics of the child. A sperm carries either an X or a Y chromosome, producing females and males respectively (see Genetics).

### The manufacture of sperm

The successful manufacture of sperm necessitates a temperature of about 1.8°F (1°C) lower than the rest of the body. Consequently, manufacture takes place outside the body, within the scrotum. Surrounding tissue helps to regulate the temperature of the testicles inside the scrotum by pulling them upward to the body in cold conditions, and by a rich supply of blood vessels which dissipate the heat when the temperature gets too high.

Sperm production—at the rate of 10 billion to 30 billion a month—takes place in the seminiferous tubules in the testicles. The newly formed sperm then pass through the seminiferous tubules into the epididymis, which is located behind the testicles. This serves as a storage and development area, the sperm taking between 60 to 72 hours to achieve full maturity. In fact, the epididymis can be emptied by three or four ejaculations in 12 hours; it takes about two days to be refilled. If ejaculation does not take place, the sperm disintegrate and are absorbed back into the bloodstream.

### Ejaculation

Before ejaculation occurs, the sperm move along the vas deferens, two tubes connecting the testicles to the prostate gland, and into a further storage area, the ampulla. Here, the sperm receive a

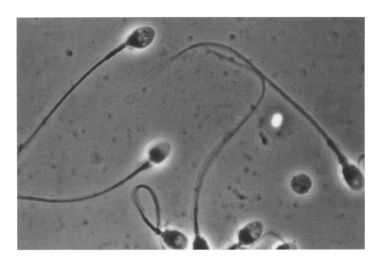

▲ *In order to reach and fertilize the female egg in the fallopian tube, the sperm must swim. Lashing their long tails is their sole method of propulsion.*

secretion from the seminal vesicles, two coiled tubes adjoining the ampulla. This secretion, called seminal fluid, stimulates the motility—the ability to move—of the sperm, and helps them survive in the vaginal secretion (see Vagina). The prostate gland, through which the sperm pass during ejaculation, produces a small amount of a similar fluid, giving the sperm full motility (see Prostate Gland).

At the moment of ejaculation, the sperm and seminal fluid are forced out of the ampullae and epididymis into the urethra by a series of muscular contractions (see Urethra). If the sperm have been ejaculated into the vagina of a woman, they move as fast as they can through the cervix and into the uterus. They then make their way into the fallopian tubes, where fertilization may occur if an egg is present.

### What can go wrong?

Fertilization is unlikely to take place if the concentration of the sperm is too low, if the sperm are abnormal in form, or if the sperm are unable to move or stop moving too soon. The condition of the seminal fluid is another vital factor, since it both nourishes and protects the sperm. Blocked tubes, infection, stress, and ill health can also cause infertility.

The number of normal, healthy sperm in one ejaculate varies widely—anything from 20 million to 350 million in the semen (the seminal fluid and the sperm together). A sperm count lower than 20 million healthy sperm may well be responsible for infertility. When infertility is suspected, a sperm specimen will be tested in a pathology lab (see Specimens), and treatment and advice will depend on the cause. A man with a low sperm count may be advised to save up his sperm for a few days so as to produce the optimum number of sperm in his ejaculate. In other cases, artificial insemination is recommended. Several ejaculations are placed in a centrifuge, and the sperm concentrate is placed on the woman's cervix at her most fertile time (see Cervix and Cervical Smears).

Doctors are unlikely to think that investigation for infertility is needed until a couple have been trying to conceive for a year or more.

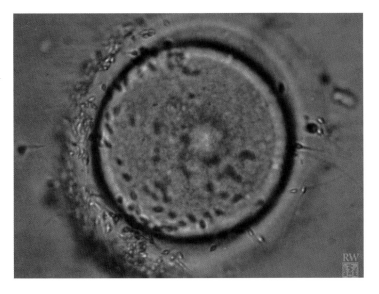

▲ *The moment of conception: chemicals in the tip of the sperm strip away the outer layer of the egg until one sperm can penetrate its smooth shell. Chemical changes in the outer layer of the egg then ensure that no further sperm can enter.*

See also: **Artificial methods of conception; Cells and chromosomes; Conception; Erection and ejaculation; Infertility; Intercourse; Puberty; Semen; Testes**

# Sphygmomanometer

## Questions and Answers

**Will it hurt to have my blood pressure taken?**

No, not at all. The most that you will feel is a tightness on your arm when the cuff is fully inflated; but this lasts for only a few seconds and amounts to mild discomfort rather than pain.

**When my blood pressure is taken I get a thumping feeling in my arm. Why?**

This is the equivalent to what the doctor hears with a stethoscope and represents the moment at which the pressure in the cuff is dropped to a point at which blood can flow into the lower arm again. It can do so only at the peak of the heart's pumping action, called systole, so you feel a thump in your arm each time your heart beats. When the pressure in the cuff is lowered again, and the blood flows freely again, the thumping disappears. The reading on the scale then represents the diastolic blood pressure.

**I understand that having your blood pressure taken involves cutting off the blood supply to one arm. Isn't this dangerous?**

No; the blood supply is cut off for only a few seconds; it would have to be interrupted for at least 10 minutes to cause damage to the tissues of the arm.

**My doctor always takes my blood pressure on the left arm, but other doctors use the other arm. Which method is correct?**

Both. Except in people with a very rare disease, the blood pressure is the same throughout the body, so it doesn't matter which arm is used. It may be that in the doctor's office, the left arm is nearest to the sphygmomanometer, so that the patient need not move.

**Our circulatory system needs a consistent pressure if it is to function efficiently. The machine used to measure this pressure is called a sphygmomanometer; it can be a mercury gauge or an aneroid device.**

The pressure of blood in the arteries fluctuates, about 80 times each minute, between a maximum that occurs at the height of the heart's contraction (the systolic pressure) and a minimum that occurs when the heart muscle relaxes between beats (the diastolic pressure). The sphygmomanometer works by comparing the pressure in the arteries with that required to support a standard column of mercury at a certain height. The familiar figures for normal blood pressure, 120/80, mean that the systolic pressure is equivalent to the force required to support a column of mercury 120 mm (4.75 inches) high, and the diastolic pressure would support a column of mercury 80 mm (3.15 inches) high. An upright glass tube (a manometer), which is graduated in millimeters and closed at the top, is connected at the bottom to a glass bulb containing mercury. It is fixed on to a backboard for support. There is an armlet or cuff for compressing the upper arm; and the rubber bulb for pumping it up is fitted with a screw valve to enable air to be released from the cuff at the right time. The three parts of the apparatus are connected by short lengths of rubber tubing. The cuff and the pressure gauge are connected so that the pressure in one is the same as the pressure in the other.

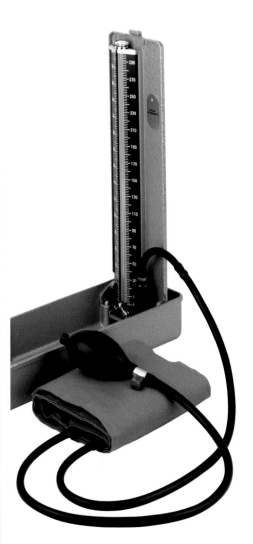

### Measuring the blood pressure

The cuff is wrapped firmly around the arm just above the elbow and the doctor pumps air into it until the pressure is sufficient to stop blood from flowing into the lower arm. He or she listens with a stethoscope over the brachial artery at the elbow. At this point the doctor will hear nothing. Continuing to listen, the doctor slightly unscrews the valve on the bulb so that air is released from the cuff and the pressure in it slowly falls. When the pressure in the cuff and in the artery are the same, the blood can flow again, but only at the systolic part of the heart's action, since the diastolic pressure is insufficient to get past the inflated cuff. The doctor will hear a series of thuds each time the heart beats and squeezes blood past the cuff. The reading on the scale then represents the systolic blood pressure (see Blood Pressure). Once the systolic level is recorded, the doctor loosens the valve further. When the thumping dies away, the reading on the scale represents the diastolic blood pressure.

▲ *Blood pressure can be measured using a mercury gauge sphygmomanometer.*

See also: **Heart; Heart disease; Kidneys and kidney diseases; Salt; Stress; Stroke**

# Spina bifida

**This serious congenital condition, which is often severely disabling, can usually be prevented. Even if it is not, however, some babies with spina bifida may be nearly normal or may be treated successfully after birth.**

## Questions and Answers

**My sister had a baby with spina bifida. Am I more likely to have a baby with this condition?**

Possibly, but the risk is quite small. Before you conceive, talk to your doctor about the importance of the B vitamin folic acid, in preventing what are now called neural tube defects. The neural tube is part of the developing embryo and is present at a very early stage. An adequate intake of folic acid at conception will greatly reduce the probability of neural tube defects. These defects in the structure of the neural tube cause the various degrees of spina bifida. As soon as you are pregnant, ask your gynecologist for a blood test to find out if the baby is healthy. Look after yourself during pregnancy. Eat a varied diet; get plenty of fresh air and suitable exercise; do not smoke or drink alcohol or take drugs. A healthy mother is more likely to have a healthy baby.

**Can a baby with spina bifida grow into a perfectly healthy adult and have healthy children?**

Yes. It depends on the severity of spina bifida with which the baby is born. If the baby is only mildly affected, then the important nerves to the legs and bladder will be undamaged. The child will develop normally and be able to have healthy children. However, adults with spina bifida do have a slightly increased risk of having a baby with spina bifida. On the other hand, if the baby is born with a severe form of the condition, he or she may have paralyzed legs and be unable to walk and will need a wheelchair. In addition, most badly affected children have poor bladder control and need to wear a special appliance to collect urine. Owing to their numerous disabilities, badly affected adults may have sexual difficulties. Nevertheless, it is possible for them to have healthy children.

Many people are confused about spina bifida because there are different types of spina bifida and the degree of disability can vary so broadly. The name "spina bifida" simply means that some of the bones in the spine have not joined properly. In fact, many people have such an abnormality without realizing it, since it causes no disabilities whatsoever.

## Possible causes

Spina bifida occurs more commonly in some families than in others. The reasons for this are not fully understood, but once an affected baby has been born, the parents, brothers, sisters, and even cousins are more likely to have an affected child than people from a family that has no history of spina bifida (see Genetics).

It has also been discovered that some mothers who have given birth to babies with spina bifida may have been lacking in the B vitamin folic acid. There is now substantial evidence that women who take a daily dose of folic acid prior to conception and during the early weeks of pregnancy will greatly reduce their likelihood of having a baby with spina bifida. The full dose required to achieve this advantage may not be provided by over-the-counter preparations, so the folic acid regimen should be prescribed by a doctor.

## Types of spina bifida

Sometimes a baby is born with a soft cyst on the back, which is called a meningocele (see Birth Defects; Cyst). The cyst usually appears on the neck or the bottom of the spine but can occur at any point and is an outward bulging of the fluid that surrounds the nerves and spinal cord. The danger is that the skin covering it may be very thin, and may become damaged and prone to infection. Early surgery is very successful in this type of spina bifida, and the baby usually grows into a perfectly normal adult.

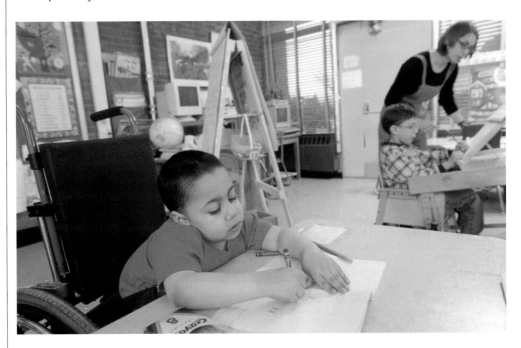

▲ *A seven-year-old boy with spina bifida is drawing in his first-grade class at the Zoller public school in Schenectady, New York.*

**I am 40 and pregnant. Do I have a greater risk of having a baby with spina bifida?**

No, not unless you have already had a baby with an abnormal brain or spine, or unless you have had several miscarriages. Statistically, however, a baby with a congenital abnormality, such as Down syndrome, is more likely to be born to a woman over 35. Both Down syndrome and spina bifida can be detected by amniocentesis, a test in which some of the amniotic fluid (the fluid surrounding the fetus) is extracted from the womb and examined. In the case of spina bifida, the amniotic fluid will contain certain chemicals in abnormal amounts.

**I had an abortion after the baby was diagnosed as having spina bifida in an amniocentesis test. Does this mean that my future pregnancies will not be normal?**

Not necessarily, but you do run a greater than average risk of conceiving another baby with a deformity of the brain or spine. However, the risk is still fairly small. If you were to have another 25 babies, it is likely that, unless you took folic acid, one would have spina bifida. The problem is that you would have no way of telling whether it would be the next one or the 25th. The only way to be sure is to have an amniocentesis with each pregnancy. Your obstetrician would probably recommend an ultrasound examination of the developing baby or even an examination of the fetus using a special viewing instrument called a fetoscope inserted into the womb. It enables the doctor to view the fetus directly. However, it would be pointless to have these tests unless you were prepared to have another termination if an abnormality were to be discovered. Before you get pregnant again, discuss folic acid with your doctor. He or she will be able to prescribe the correct dose, since the vitamin must be taken in adequate dosage to achieve the fullest protection.

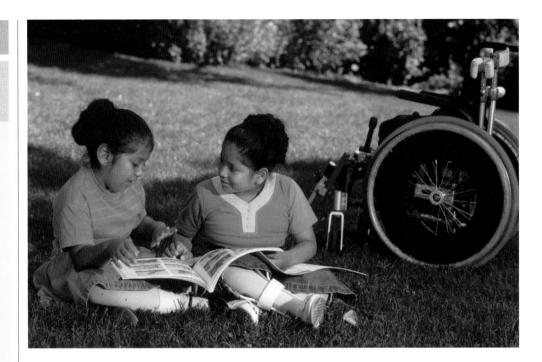

▲ *Children with disabilities and those without disabilities are happy to play and learn together without any inhibitions.*

Most cases of spina bifida, however, are more serious. A baby born with open spina bifida, for example, has part of the backbone, some nerves, and the spinal cord lying exposed at the bottom of the cyst, which often bursts even before birth. Most babies with this type of spina bifida will have disabilities, the severity of which depends on the part of the back affected and the amount of damage to nerves. Since the extent of nerve damage varies greatly, the baby may have little or no disability or, at the other extreme, may be severely disabled. If the neck is affected, then the nerves used for breathing are usually damaged, and nearly all these babies die soon after birth.

If the base of the spine is involved, only a few nerves going to the feet may be abnormal and the baby can be born with nothing more serious than clubfoot (see Clubfoot). This can be cured by physical therapy (see Physical Therapy), which the mother can be taught so that she can treat the baby herself at home, or by orthopedic surgery. Sometimes a few of the nerves that control the bladder are slightly damaged, so that the child may have poor bladder control (see Incontinence).

If the middle of the back is affected, the results are more serious. Generally, the higher the opening in the back, the worse the outlook. Children affected in this way will have at least some deformity or weakness of the legs; some will never be able to walk and will have to use a wheelchair. Others will be able to walk after repeated surgery on their bones and tendons, if they wear braces for support (see Orthopedics).

Many of these children are incontinent of bowel and bladder and may need some form of incontinence control such as a catheter to drain the urine. A severely affected child may also develop curvature of the spine at puberty;

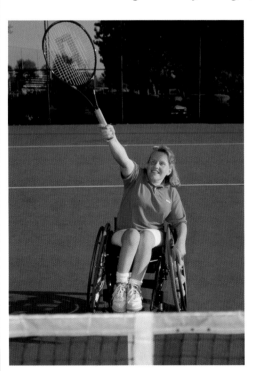

▲ *Gina Jalbert is an expert tennis player, despite having spina bifida.*

## TWO TYPES OF SPINA BIFIDA

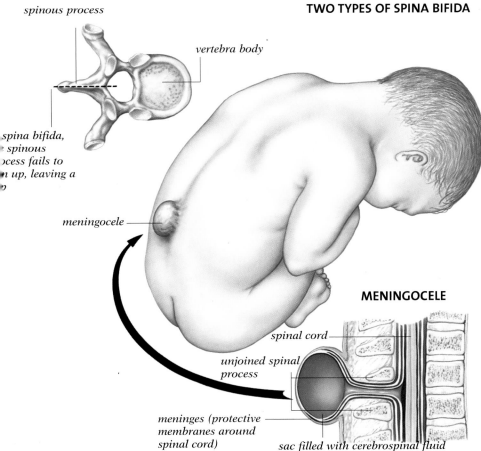

*spinous process*

*vertebra body*

*spina bifida, spinous cess fails to n up, leaving a*

*meningocele*

**MENINGOCELE**

*spinal cord*

*unjoined spinal process*

*meninges (protective membranes around spinal cord)*

*sac filled with cerebrospinal fluid*

**MYELOMENINGOCELE**

*vertebral body*

*spinal cord*

*cerebrospinal fluid*

*nerves*

*unjoined spinous process*

*In spina bifida, the two halves of the spinous process (which normally forms the vertebral arch) fail to join up. A baby may then be born with a meningocele, a cyst over a gap in the spine that contains spinal fluid. This can be treated by surgery on the newborn baby. A more serious form is the myelomeningocele, in which some nerves and the spinal cord are exposed, and bones may even be missing. This always causes a degree of paralysis.*

this problem can, however, be rectified by major surgery. Hydrocephalus (excessive water in the brain) often accompanies this type of spina bifida. The fluid has to be drained out into the chest or abdomen through special tubes and valves. In another form of spina bifida the baby is born apparently healthy except for a fatty lump at the bottom of the back. The danger of this is that it may be ignored because the baby can move his or her legs when newly born. However, this condition may deteriorate as the child gets older, so it is very important that a specialist sees him or her for regular checkups. Surgery may be undertaken to free the nerves at the first sign of trouble, though this is not always successful.

### Possible treatments

An expert should examine a baby born with spina bifida immediately, even though this may mean that the baby has to be separated from the mother and sent to a special facility, where he or she will be in the care of a pediatric surgeon (see Pediatrics).

A whole team of specialists can then decide whether or not the baby will benefit from surgery, which is often carried out before the baby is 24 hours old in order to achieve the best results as well as to reduce the risk of serious infection. Many surgeons will not recommend surgery if it is thought that the baby will grow up with severe deformities, lack of bladder control, and hydrocephalus.

If the baby cannot be helped by urgent surgery, then doctors may differ in their advice to parents. Some doctors recommend that the parents take the baby home as soon as they feel able to cope. Many of these babies die from meningitis within a few weeks. However, the others feed well and the spina bifida heals by itself in about six

to eight weeks, although it frequently forms a large cyst, which has to be removed several months later. Many of these babies develop fluid on the brain, which has to be treated surgically when they are three to six months old. Alternatively, some doctors think that they are best kept in a hospital to be given regular painkillers. Severely affected babies do not feed well and most die within six months. The difficult decision rests with the parents to decide the kind of treatment they want their baby to have. Parents who care for their baby at home may find it helpful to contact one of the spina bifida associations, which can give support.

### Prevention

For most new babies, spina bifida is now a defect that is very unlikely to occur. Research published in 1989 as well as several later studies showed conclusively that the risk of spina bifida can be greatly reduced if a small daily intake of folic acid is taken before pregnancy starts and during early pregnancy. The dose needed is no more than 0.4 mg per day, but for women who have already had a baby with spina bifida, a much larger dose is required. The folic acid must be taken at the time the neural tube is forming. This occurs early, so the vitamin should be taken before the pregnancy starts. It has been found that folic acid supplements do not increase the risk of miscarriage. In 1998, legislation was passed requiring folic acid to be added to bread and pasta; since then, the incidence of spina bifida in the United States has declined by almost 20 percent.

*See also:* **Hydrocephalus; Meningitis; Scoliosis**

# Spinal cord

**Is the spinal column always damaged by a broken neck?**

Not always, but often; yet the spinal cord can be injured without there being a fracture of the spinal bones. This tends to happen when the cord is suddenly stretched or twisted in an accident. More important than the fracture is whether any bones are displaced, causing them to press onto the cord in the spinal canal that runs through the spinal bones.

**Is it true that ordinary viruses, such as those that cause flu, can cause an infection of the spinal cord?**

This type of myelitis can occur, but it is rare. It's probable that those who are attacked by a virus in this way have some subtle abnormality of their immunity defenses at the time of exposure to the virus. The virus invades the body; afterward there appears to be some form of reaction between the immune system and the virus, with the result that nervous tissue in the spine is damaged. Poliomyelitis is rather different, since it is caused by one of three related viruses. The virus invades the motor cells of the spinal cord and parts of the brain, and disrupts the motor signals from the brain to the muscles.

**My friend has multiple sclerosis and has a lot of trouble controlling her bladder. Why should this be?**

The urge to urinate is controlled by a reflex action of the brain; when the bladder is full, sensations pass to the brain telling us that the bladder desperately needs to be emptied. In multiple sclerosis, nerve damage impairs the passage of information. In some cases, sensations of a full bladder do not reach the brain, and in others the messages from the brain telling the bladder sphincter to remain shut do not reach the sphincter. The outcome is usually incontinence.

**A vital link in the nervous system, the spinal cord gathers and analyzes information from the body and channels it to and from the brain. When this link is damaged or broken, however, permanent disability may result.**

The spinal cord runs down most of the length of the bony part of the spine. It forms a vital link between the brain and the nerves connected to the rest of the body. However, the spinal cord is far more than simply a bundle of nerve fibers that go to and from the brain. It acts as an important initial analyzer for incoming sensations, and as a programming station for organizing some of the basic movements of the limbs.

## SPINAL CORD

▼ *The spinal cord is protected by cerebrospinal fluid and membranes, and runs from the brain to the second lumbar vertebra before tapering into the filum terminale. A cross section of the cord (top right) shows sensory and motor pathways carrying messages to and from the brain. Reflex action occurs when messages cross the connector nerve.*

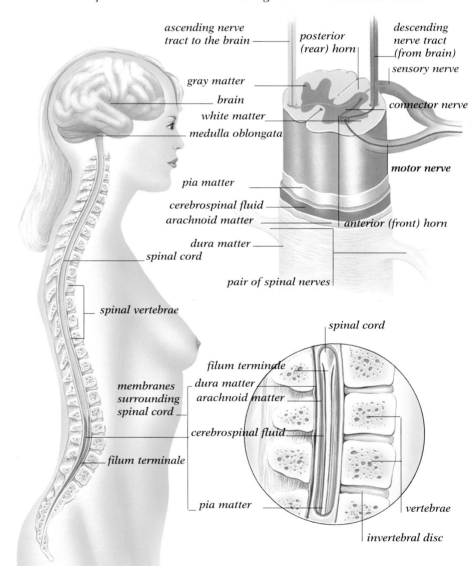

A number of conditions can affect the spinal cord, and injuries to this delicate structure can be devastating. The physical effects of any injury depend on which part of the cord is damaged, or which parts of it take the brunt of the injury.

## Structure of the spinal cord

The spinal cord runs from the medulla oblongata in the brain stem down to the first or second lumbar vertebra.

The cord is well protected as it passes through the arches of the spinal vertebrae. Sensory and motor nerves of the peripheral nervous system leave the spinal cord separately just below the vertebrae and then join to form 31 pairs of spinal nerves (eight cervical, 12 thoracic, five lumbar, five sacral, and one coccygeal), each nerve corresponding to the vertebra that it leaves. These nerves branch out from the spinal cord, spreading to the surface of the body and to all the skeletal muscles (see Muscles).

The spinal cord is composed of collections of nerve cell bodies: neurons and bundles of nerve fibers. The gray matter, or the nerve cell collections, is H-shaped in cross section, with a posterior (rear) and anterior (front) horn (protuberance) in each half. The anterior is composed of motor neurons; the posterior horn contains cell bodies of connector neurons and sensory neurons.

The gray matter is surrounded by the white matter. The white matter is divided into columns and contains ascending and descending nerve tracts which connect the brain and the spinal cord in both directions. The descending tracts send motor impulses from the brain to the peripheral nervous system; the ascending tracts channel sensory impulses to the brain.

Surrounding these nerves and fibers is a series of membranes which are extensions of those membranes that surround the brain (see Membranes). Between the outer two of these three membrane layers is a small gap which contains cerebrospinal fluid. This circulates around the spinal cord and the brain, providing nutrients to the nerves and acting as a protective buffer.

## Functions of the spinal cord

The spinal cord has two main functions: to act as a two-way conduction system between the brain and the peripheral nervous system, and to control simple reflex actions (see Reflexes).

The spinal cord and the brain make up the central nervous system. Messages, in the form of electrical impulses created by the firing of interconnected neurons, from the surface of the body connect with the spinal cord via the sensory nerve fibers in the peripheral nervous system. The gray matter in the spinal cord rapidly processes the messages, and then relays some of them up the ascending tract of the spinal cord for more detailed analysis in the brain.

If some action is required, the brain sends messages of action, in the form of motor impulses, down the descending tract that result in coordinated muscular action involving many different muscles in the body.

For example, when an itch is felt in the hand (see Itches), initial analysis takes place at the spinal cord. Further analysis then takes place in the brain, which may then send messages in response, instructing the appropriate muscles of the body to move accordingly.

In controlling the simple reflex action the usual pattern of message transmission to the brain is drastically curtailed. If the skin touches something hot, streams of impulses are passed via the sensory neurons to the posterior horn in the gray matter of the spinal cord. Instead of then ascending to the brain, the messages are immediately processed, and then cross to the anterior horn of the gray matter via connector neurons. These allow messages to be transmitted from sensory neurons to motor neurons, giving an immediate physical response—the hand is rapidly and automatically withdrawn. This is known as the reflex arc. At the same time, information will be passed on to the brain, which will determine further action, if any.

Many of the body's important functions are controlled through reflex action and these occur at all levels of the spinal cord. Some movements involved in respiration, digestion, and especially excretion, for example, are reflex actions controlled in part by the spinal cord (see Autonomic Nervous System).

## Spinal cord problems

A variety of conditions can seriously affect the spinal cord, from those that are acquired before birth, such as spina bifida, to others that can appear later on in life, like multiple sclerosis.

**Spina bifida:** In this fairly common type of birth defect, the spine and the spinal cord fail to develop normally in the womb. A flat plate of cells on the embryo's back normally folds itself into a tube, which then develops into the spine and spinal cord. In spina bifida,

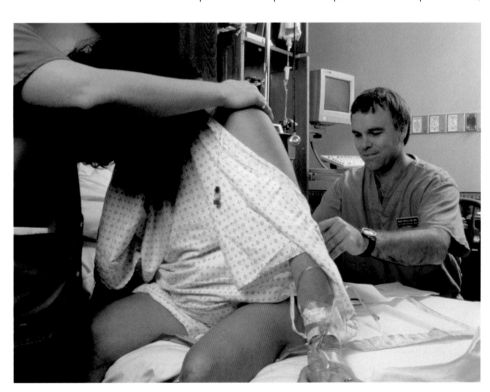

▲ *A woman receives an epidural—an injection of painkilling medication into the epidermal area between the dura mater and the more interior regions of the spinal cord—to ease her labor pains in the hospital delivery room during childbirth.*

## Questions and Answers

**In a spinal tap, is the fluid taken off through the needle from the spinal cord itself? If so, isn't there a risk of damage to the cord?**

The spinal cord ends about three-quarters of the way down the spine. The spinal canal (the space enclosed by the bones of the spine), which is below that, is only partly filled by the nerves which go down to the legs. So there is room for a needle to remove fluid without damaging the nerves. The fluid is the same as that which circulates around the brain and through the center of the cord, so it is useful to examine in diagnosing conditions affecting the nervous system.

**Are the cells of the spinal cord like brain cells or are they different?**

The nerve cells, or neurons, of the spinal cord are the same as those of the brain. Although some are specialized for their particular job (like some brain cells) they are essentially the same.

**I have heard that the spinal cord is affected by syphilis. Is this true?**

This is now uncommon, but one of the delayed effects of syphilis can be to attack the sensory nerves just as they are entering the spinal cord. This causes the rear part of the cord, which is made up of the sensory fibers on their way to the brain, to wither. The main symptom from the loss of these nerves is a poor sense of where the joints are, making walking difficult.

**Is the spinal cord always seriously deformed when a baby is born with spina bifida?**

No, the spinal cord is not always deformed. There are degrees of severity. It is only in the most severe type that the spinal cord is involved and the bone fails to fold over as it should as the baby develops in the womb. Sometimes spina bifida involves only the bones of the spine, and there is seldom any spinal cord trouble.

## AREAS OF THE BODY CONTROLLED BY THE SPINAL NERVES

► *The majority of signals that control the body's sensations and movement are fed to and from the brain via the 31 pairs of nerves joining the spinal column. These nerves control different areas of the body. If the cord is damaged, all areas fed by the nerves below the site of the injury will be affected.*

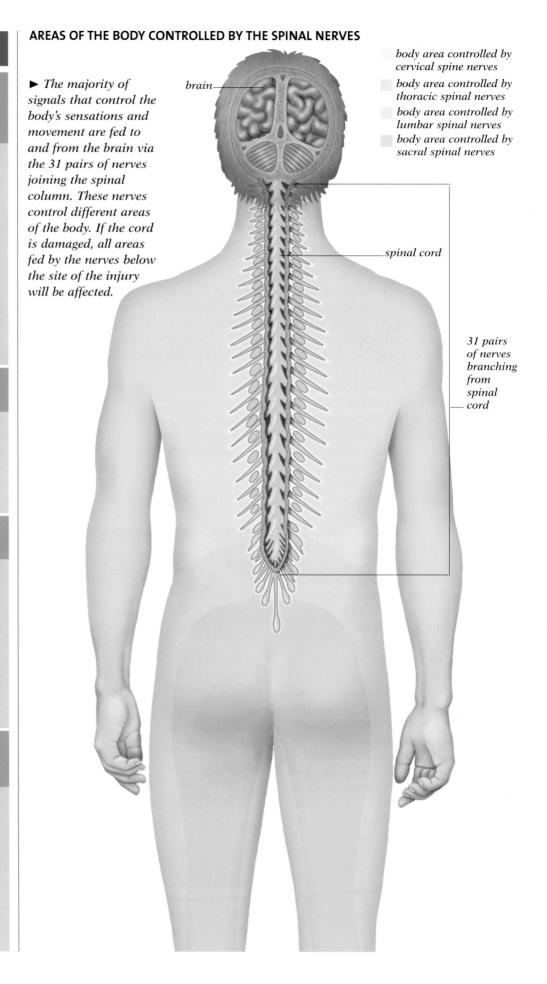

- body area controlled by cervical spine nerves
- body area controlled by thoracic spinal nerves
- body area controlled by lumbar spinal nerves
- body area controlled by sacral spinal nerves

brain

spinal cord

*31 pairs of nerves branching from spinal cord*

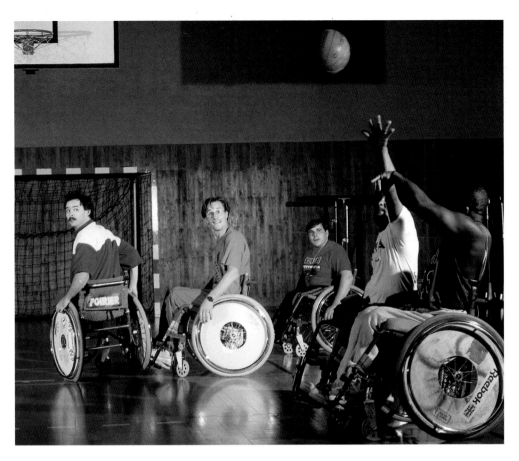

▲ *Competitive sports like basketball are actively pursued and enjoyed by many people with severe spinal injuries. Differing degrees of mobility and expertise can be achieved.*

**Tumors:** These rarely occur inside the spinal cord itself, but the cord can be pressed on by tumors from the outside. The effects of this type of complaint on the cord, and what symptoms are produced, depend on where the tumor is located. Occasional pains around the trunk, or down an arm or leg, are common symptoms of a tumor pressing on the nerves emerging from the cord. Sensation may also be lost from either side of the body below the site of the trouble. As with spinal injuries, the person may also become incontinent (see Incontinence).

Treatment depends on where the tumor is located, but it usually involves either surgical removal of the tumor or drainage of the abscess. In the case of a cancerous tumor, radiotherapy may be used (see Radiotherapy; Tumors).

**Multiple sclerosis:** The cause of this type of inflammation is still unknown. It attacks nerve tissue anywhere in the body, particularly the main nerves to the eye, the optic nerve, and nerves in the brain stem and the spinal cord, especially in the neck area. Spinal cord damage from multiple sclerosis can cause progressive loss of sensation and occasional tingling feelings in the hands and feet (see Multiple Sclerosis).

however, this process is disrupted, leaving the spinal cord malformed and exposed at the back.

The condition may leave the child with complete paralysis of the legs and no control over either urination or defecation. In some severe cases, brain damage may also occur (see Brain Damage and Disease). The type of treatment that may be possible will depend on how badly deformed the spinal cord is (see Spina Bifida).

**Injuries to the spinal cord:** This is the most common cause of problems with the spinal cord, displaced vertebrae and whiplash injuries being the most frequent types of injury (see Whiplash Injury).

Exactly what functions are lost is determined by which part of the spinal cord is actually damaged. If the cord is damaged high in the neck, all the limbs will be paralyzed (this condition is known as quadriplegia), and there may even be difficulty in breathing. Immediately after the injury all the limbs become limp, with all feeling being lost below the level of the injury. In addition, bladder control is considerably affected. After a period of weeks or months, various changes appear in the paralyzed legs and arms, as the spinal cord below the injury recovers a little. The limbs become stiff and may respond briskly with reflex movements. In some cases, there may be more improvement, and the injured person may even achieve a stiff-legged walk. If the injury is in the middle of the back, then only the legs are affected (this condition is known as paraplegia). The bladder's function is usually affected in any spinal cord injury, since the nerves to the bladder leave the cord at its lower end (see Bladder and Bladder Problems). Sexual function is lost, too, because the nerves involved are also located at the lower end.

**Myelitis:** This term means inflammation of the spinal cord (see Inflammation), and so includes multiple sclerosis. However, myelitis can be caused by some common viruses, when there is only one attack (see Viruses), unlike the repetitive attacks which characterize multiple sclerosis. The cord becomes acutely inflamed at a particular spot; below this, all function may be lost. This form of myelitis may follow an attack of flu, or some other trivial form of viral infection (see Guillan-Barré Syndrome).

**Vitamin deficiency:** A lack of the vitamin B12 can produce a particular pattern of damage to the spinal cord (as well as to the peripheral nerves). The parts of the spinal cord affected include the muscle running down the side of the cord and the sensory nerves which convey sensations of touch and a sense of where the joints are.

The affected person may suffer from a mild weakness in the limbs and have an odd, high-stepping walk because the person has difficulty in establishing where the feet are in relation to his or her body. Some recovery from this condition can be brought about when the vitamin deficiency is treated (see Vitamin B).

Many conditions affecting the spinal cord are long-term problems; recovery, if any, is slow and painstaking, and the patient will require devoted nursing. Recovery from a spinal cord injury may never be complete, especially if the damage is severe, but considerable movement and control can be regained through regular exercise.

*See also:* **Bones; Brain; Neck; Nervous system; Paralysis; Paraplegia; Poliomyelitis; Skeleton; Spina bifida**

# Spleen

**I've heard that the spleen can burst during glandular fever. Is this true, and is it dangerous?**

It is possible, but it is a very rare occurrence. If the spleen bursts as a result of the glandular fever virus, then its contents will be released into the abdomen where they may inflame the membrane lining the abdomen, and give rise to peritonitis. A burst spleen can be dangerous, but it happens very infrequently.

**My brother insists that he has two spleens. Can this be true?**

Yes. There is usually only one big spleen to be found in the abdomen, normally in the top left-hand corner, but occasionally there may be one or two accessory spleens in the same general area.

**A friend of mine had to have his spleen removed after a traffic accident. Does this mean that his blood will be affected?**

The spleen plays a major part in ridding the body of harmful bacteria and in making antibodies, so its removal makes a person, particularly a child, more susceptible to serious bacterial infections. Some physicians recommend prophylactic antibiotic treatment for all postsplenectomy patients.

**Does the spleen influence a person's emotional state?**

No. It was once thought that the spleen was the seat of anger, and morose people were said to have a splenic personality. We still talk of venting our spleen, which means to get angry, but there is no scientific basis for this. No one knows why a blood-forming and blood-filtering organ should have acquired this reputation.

**Situated in the top left-hand corner of the abdomen, the spleen plays a major role in blood formation and influences the development of immunity. In addition, it may signal disease elsewhere in the body.**

The spleen is an important organ of the body. Its main function is to filter the blood and to make antibodies. An enlarged spleen, which can be felt through the walls of the abdomen, is often an indication of disease somewhere in the body. The spleen is also an integral part of the lymphatic system—the basis of the body's defense against infection.

## Location

The spleen lies just below the diaphragm at the top of the left-hand side of the abdomen. It is normally about 5 inches (13 cm) long, and it lies along the line of the tenth rib. The spleen usually weighs about ½ pound (about 200 g) in adults, but, in cases where it is enlarged, it can weigh up to 4½ pounds (2 kg) or more.

## Appearance

If a spleen is examined with the naked eye, it will look like a fibrous capsule surrounding a mass of featureless red pulp. It may just be possible to make out little granulations called Malpighian corpuscles. The organ is supplied with blood via the splenic artery, which, like any other artery,

### POSITION OF THE SPLEEN

*The spleen is situated in the top left-hand corner of the abdomen, just below the diaphragm. It is in a relatively exposed position, and so it is frequently damaged in accidents and has to be removed, generally without any ill effects.*

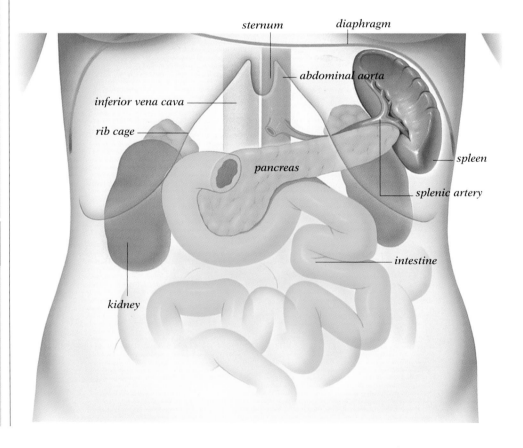

sternum · diaphragm · abdominal aorta · inferior vena cava · rib cage · pancreas · spleen · splenic artery · intestine · kidney

splits first into smaller arteries and then into tiny arterioles. However, the arterioles of the spleen are unusual in that they are wrapped in lymphatic tissue as they pass through the pulp of the spleen. The arterioles are unique in another way; instead of being connected to a network of capillaries, they appear to empty out into the main mass of the spleen.

The unusual way in which the spleen is supplied with blood is what enables it to perform two of its basic functions. First, the fact that the arterioles are wrapped with lymphatic tissue means that the lymphatic system comes into immediate contact with any abnormal protein in the blood and forms antibodies to it. Second, the way that the blood empties directly into the pulp of the spleen also allows the reticular cells of the organ to come into direct contact with the blood, filtering it of any old or worn-out cells.

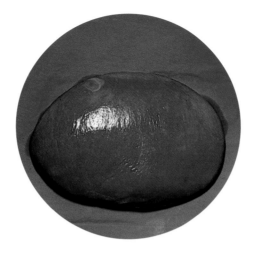

▲ *The healthy spleen is an organ that usually weighs about ½ lb. (200 g) in adults and is 5 in. (13 cm) long.*

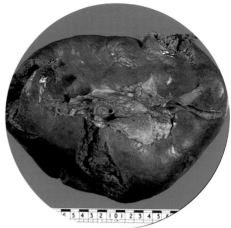

▲ *A diseased spleen: this spleen is greatly enlarged because of the presence of a lymphoma or lymphatic tumor.*

## Functions of the spleen

The spleen is one of the main filters of the blood. Not only do the reticular cells remove old and worn-out blood cells, but they will also remove any abnormal cells. This applies, in particular, to red blood cells, but white cells and platelets are also filtered selectively when necessary by the spleen (see Blood).

The spleen will also remove abnormal particles floating in the bloodstream. This means that it plays a major part in ridding the body of harmful bacteria. It is also instrumental in making antibodies—proteins circulating in the blood that will bind onto and immobilize a foreign protein so that white blood cells called phagocytes can destroy it. The Malpighian corpuscles, which are collections of lymphocytes, produce the antibody.

In some circumstances, the spleen has an important role in the manufacture of new blood cells. This does not happen in the normal adult, but in people who have a bone marrow disease the spleen and the liver are major sites of red blood cell production. In addition, the spleen makes a large proportion of the blood of an unborn baby.

## Feeling the spleen

The spleen cannot be felt in normal healthy people, but there is a large range of diseases that cause enlargement of the spleen, which can then be felt through the walls of the abdomen. The procedure is that the patient lies on his or her back, and the doctor starts to feel (or palpate) the bottom of the abdomen, and then works up toward the top left-hand corner. The spleen moves as the patient breathes, so he or she is asked to take deep breaths so that this movement can be felt. Enlargement of the spleen can also be detected on X rays or by using a radioactive isotope scan.

## Enlargement of the spleen

The spleen may enlarge for many reasons. Since one of its main functions is to break down old and worn-out blood cells, those conditions where blood is broken down faster than normal are associated with an enlarged spleen. These diseases are called hemolytic anemias, and many of them, such as sickle-cell anemia (see Sickle-Cell Anemia) or thalassemia (see Thalassemia), are inherited. Hemolytic problems can also have other causes; for example, some drugs such as methyldopa (used to control blood pressure) may cause hemolysis and thus a large spleen. Other blood diseases also cause the spleen to become enlarged. In some

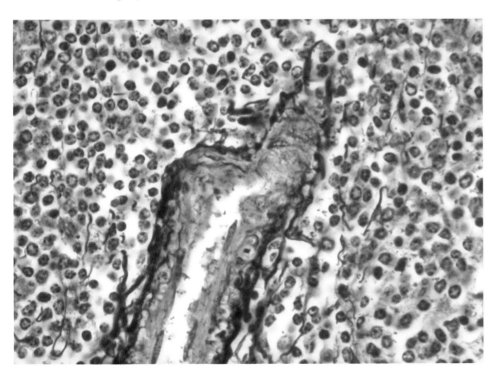

▲ *Spleen tissue, which is the site of phagocytosis and initiation of immune responses, is shown stained and magnified 160 times.*

## GEOGRAPHICAL DISTRIBUTION OF KALA-AZAR

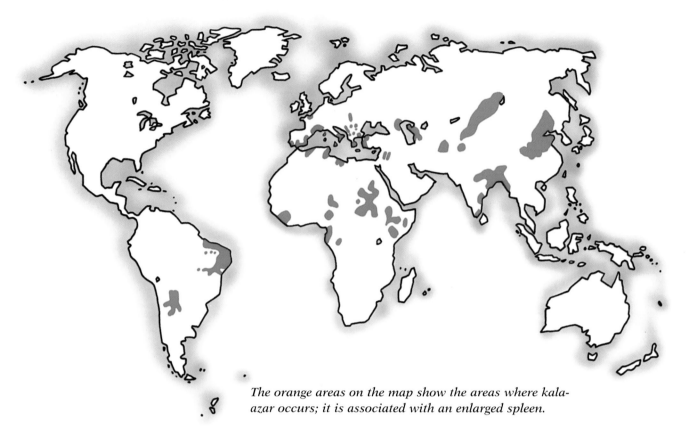

*The orange areas on the map show the areas where kala-azar occurs; it is associated with an enlarged spleen.*

cases of leukemia, for example, the spleen grows so much that it stretches from the top left-hand corner of the abdomen to the bottom right-hand corner (see Leukemia).

There are two other diseases that are associated with an enlarged spleen, malaria and the parasitic disease called kala-azar, in which the parasites actually inhabit the spleen. Because it is involved in the body's immune mechanisms against infection, many other infections can cause an enlarged spleen. A common disease associated with the enlargement of the spleen is glandular fever. Occasionally, the large spleen found in this illness can rupture as a result of a comparatively minor injury to the abdomen, and an operation will be needed.

The veins of the spleen drain into the portal system of veins. These are the veins that drain blood that is rich with nutrients from the intestines into the liver. Thus, when liver disease is present, pressure on the system can rise, putting pressure on the spleen, which enlarges. Thus, an enlarged spleen can indicate that there is trouble in the liver. Also, it is a useful indicator of health of the body, since its enlargement may be a result of problems elsewhere. Little can go wrong with the spleen; cysts and benign tumors may form rarely.

### Removal of the spleen

There are, however, a number of reasons why the spleen may have to be removed.

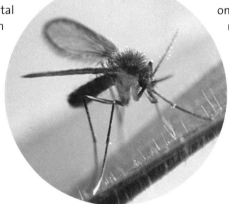

▲ *Kala-azar is caused by the bite of some sand flies; if the right treatment is not available, it can be fatal.*

Despite the fact that it is an important filter of the blood, very few immediate effects seem to result from its removal. The susceptibility to severe infections is, however, increased.

If the spleen should rupture or become injured as the result of an accident, it tends to bleed profusely; the only option then is to surgically remove it. The spleen may also have to be removed during laparotomies (investigative operations during which the abdomen is opened) in order to investigate the extent of lymphomas or lymphatic tumors (see Cancer; Lymphoma).

Occasionally the spleen becomes overactive in its function of breaking down blood cells, and this overactivity leads to excessive destruction of cells. This is likely to happen only when the spleen is already enlarged for some reason, such as a lymphoma or portal hypertension due to liver disease. In these cases, too, the spleen may be removed.

The spleen is therefore a unique organ; for whereas it has useful and straightforward functions, the body seems capable of functioning quite well without a spleen. Another anomaly is that although the spleen rarely malfunctions, it is an indicator of problems, and it is often involved in other defects elsewhere in the body.

*See also:* **Infectious mononucleosis; Liver and liver diseases; Malaria**

# Splinters

## Questions and Answers

**How should splinters or fragments in the eye be dealt with?**

Splinters in the eye must be treated with great care because the danger of causing further damage is considerable and could have serious results. First, stop the patient from rubbing his or her eye. Second, flood the eye with a steady flow of water, at the same time getting the patient to blink rapidly. If the object is on the center of the eye and does not come away with washing, make no further attempt to remove it. Take the patient to the hospital as soon as possible. If the splinter is not visible, sit down facing the patient and slowly draw the lower eyelid outward and downward while he or she looks up. If you still do not see it, check under the upper eyelid, with the person looking down. When you see the object, try removing it using the corner of a clean handkerchief. If it does not come away easily, do not persist, and never use tweezers to dislodge the splinter. Again, take the patient to the hospital so that a doctor can deal with the problem.

**How should fishhooks embedded in the skin be removed?**

First, clean the area with soap and water, and apply disinfectant. Never try to drag the hook, which is barbed, back through the skin. In fact, push it further forward until the point and the barb come out through the skin again. Using pliers or wire-cutters cut through the shaft of the hook. Remove the eye and the attached line. Grip the hook firmly and pull it out of the second hole in the skin.

**What should you put on a splinter wound, and should it be covered?**

Use a clean dressing or adhesive bandage to cover the wound, to stop it from getting dirty.

**Getting a splinter is a very common experience and usually it is trivial. However, since an untreated splinter can cause infection or damage to the tissues, it should always be dealt with promptly.**

Although splinters are normally pieces of wood, they can also consist of some other material, such as glass or metal.

## Why splinters can be harmful

Splinters may damage some underlying structure such as an artery or nerve by puncturing it. This is much more likely to happen with large metal splinters, which can enter the body with considerable force and penetrate deeply. A splinter can form a focus for infection; an inevitable result is that germs are instantly transported through the body's defensive covering of skin and affect the underlying tissue where conditions are ideal for germ reproduction (see Bacteria).

## Treatment

Large splinters, or splinters that have gone deep into the flesh, should be left undisturbed until they have been seen by a doctor. Even if there is a large piece of glass protruding from a wound, it must be left alone. It has done all the damage it is going to do for the time being. If a splinter has penetrated the wall of a major artery, it may be effectively plugging the wound; attempting to pull it out could potentially cause a massive hemorrhage. In addition, if the splinter is very jagged, far more damage could be caused by dragging it out.

When a splinter can be seen clearly and safely removed without risk of causing further damage, removal can be attempted by anyone competent. If it is sticking out from under the skin or a nail, the affected part should be held firmly with one hand, the splinter should be gripped as close to the site of entry as possible with tweezers, then it can be pulled out in one firm movement. The end of a splinter must never be pulled; the splinter is likely to break or the tweezers may slip.

To deal with a splinter that is completely embedded, a long, fine needle is sterilized by holding the sharp end in a flame for 10 seconds. The point can be used to open up the track of the splinter from the tail toward the point of entry, so that the splinter can be lifted out with tweezers. Opening the track from the point of entry downward may drive it further in and trying to lift it from the side is likely to break it. After removal, the wound should be sterilized with antiseptic and covered with a dressing, or an antiseptic cream can be left on for 24 hours.

▲ *Getting a splinter can be a painful and upsetting experience. Parents should err on the side of caution and seek help if a splinter cannot be removed easily.*

**See also: Infection and infectious diseases; Lacerations; Nails; Wounds**

# Splints

## Questions and Answers

**Can applying a splint to a broken leg do more harm than good?**

An incorrectly fitted splint can be very dangerous. If it is applied too tightly to the limb, circulation may be impaired. A broken leg swells rapidly after injury, so a splint that was initially safe may become too tight. Also, any sharp edges of the splint may dig into the flesh and cause a blister or sore. If you have to put a splint on a broken leg, make sure you know what you're doing. Better yet, if possible, wait for someone who is qualified to do it.

**Are splints used for all types of fractures, even hairline ones?**

Splints are used mainly when the fracture is unstable, that is, it is able to move around. Hairline fractures are usually stable, since they are held firm by surrounding tissues. Splinting isn't necessary and can even be harmful. Rib fractures, for example, are no longer splinted, since splinting makes breathing difficult.

**What is the difference between a splint and a brace?**

A brace is a type of splint. It is more sophisticated in that it may have hinges or springs to allow certain joints to move while preventing others from moving. Braces are used for long-term problems and are therefore made of very strong, durable materials.

**I saw a paramedic applying what looked like a plastic bag to a broken leg. What was this?**

An inflatable splint, a clear, heavy plastic bag shaped roughly like a leg that opens along the top with a zipper. The injured leg is placed in the bag, which is inflated, giving good all-around support. Such splints are only temporary.

**Although most often used on limbs, splints can act as external supports for any injured part of the body. Splints range from simple wooden strips to highly sophisticated devices such as braces.**

A splint is an external support for an injured or wounded part of the body. Splints can be used for various injuries, but are most commonly employed on the limbs. They can vary from simple wooden strips bandaged to a fractured bone to complicated devices with hinges, springs, and buckles. Casts, supports, and braces are all different types of splint.

## Uses of splints

**Fractures and sprains:** Splints have several functions in the treatment of fractures and sprains. First, the splint protects an injured limb from further damage by providing a hard casing in the form of a cast and by stopping movement. Second, the splint holds the limb rigid in a particular position. This is an important function because once the fracture has begun to heal it is essential that the bone is held firmly and knits together in the correct place without deformity. Third, the splint may allow the fractured limb to be used while the injury is healing (see Fractures; Sprains).

**Childhood disorders:** In some childhood conditions, certain parts of the body do not grow or develop properly because they are in the wrong position. The best example is congenital dislocation of the hip. In this condition, a splint may be used to keep the hip joint in position while it undergoes a period of growth, at the same time allowing the infant some freedom of movement, as well as giving a parent access for changing diapers and washing (see Hip).

**Paralytic conditions:** In these conditions, splints are used either to take over the function of paralyzed muscles, or to prevent joints from becoming deformed by the abnormal pull of the muscles. These splints are complicated, since they often need to be joined to allow easy

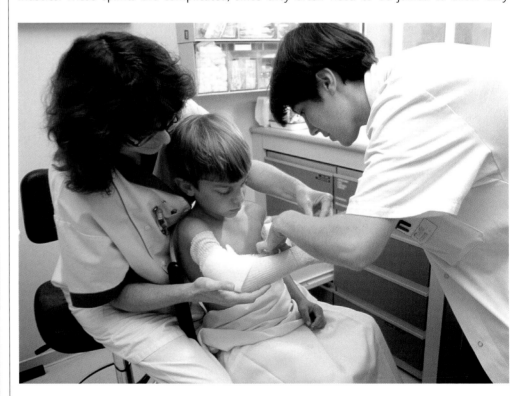

▲ *A boy having a plaster cast put on his broken arm. The cast is actually a bandage wound round and left to set. It supports the limb while the break is healing.*

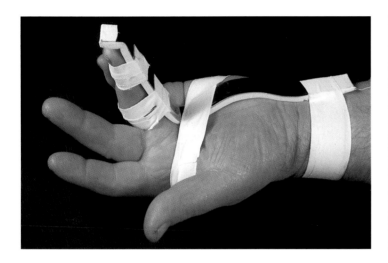

▲ *A finger splint will hold a broken bone in the correct position until it is healed, and prevent deformity.*

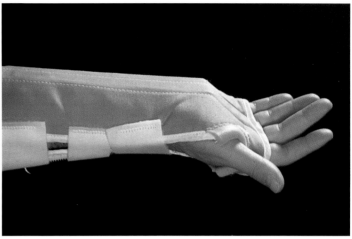

▲ *An arm splint and brace will hold the limb rigidly in position until the fracture heals.*

movement, and should be able to be removed easily. They may also incorporate springs to back up weak or paralyzed muscles.

**Arthritis:** Temporary splints may be useful in resting joints afflicted with acute arthritis. They may also be used to correct severe deformity (see Arthritis).

## What are splints made of?

The most simple and widely used splinting material is plaster of paris. Most common fractures that require splints are set in a cast made of bandage material that is impregnated with plaster powder. When the roll of plaster bandage is dipped in water it can then be molded closely to the injured limb in the few minutes that it takes for the cast to dry. Once dry, the cast is strong and durable. However,

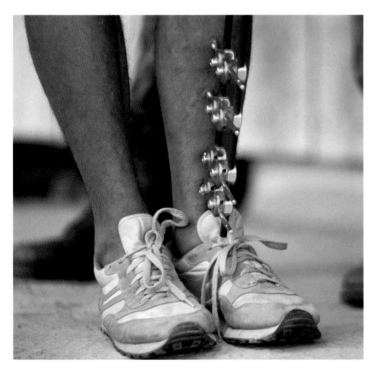

▲ *This man's fractured leg is held together by an external metal rod splint with pins inserted through the skin.*

it is heavy and can soften if it becomes wet. Resin casts are also used and are applied in the same way as a plaster cast, that is, as a bandage. They have the advantage of being light, waterproof and hard-wearing, and do not restrict the blood supply to the limb.

Newer plastic materials have been developed to overcome the disadvantages of plaster. Simple plastic sheets, which become pliable when they are heated, can be molded to fit a limb. These tend to be softer than plaster and are particularly useful when a splint has to be replaced frequently.

Splints needed for longer-term use, however, continue to be made of leather and metal. Leg braces, for example, need to fit snugly and comfortably, and yet must be strong and resilient enough to withstand the repeated stresses of walking. Leather braces have not yet been surpassed by synthetic versions: leather is strong and soft and, unlike plastic, it is permeable to moisture, so it prevents the skin from becoming damp.

Splints may be used temporarily or permanently. A splint may be employed as an interim first-aid measure for transporting an injured person to the hospital. Casts for treating fractures will have to be worn for two weeks to several months. Some people may have to wear a splint permanently to stabilize a weak limb.

### Dangers

Any rigid device fixed to the body involves certain risks. The most obvious is that the device may rub and chafe on the skin and cause a blister or sore (see Blisters; Sores). A splint that encircles the limb is potentially more dangerous. If, for example, a limb swells when it is encased in a cast, the cast will compress the limb and may eventually damage its blood supply and nerve supply. For this reason, most hospitals will require a patient to return the day after the fracture has been set to make sure that the cast is safe and comfortable. In addition, the first cast put on a fracture may be split so that if the limb swells the cast can be widened.

Another danger is that joints immobilized by a splint may become stiff. When the splint is removed they will need time to loosen up, and physical therapy or exercises are usually necessary.

*See also:* **Bones; Exercise; Physical therapy; Skeleton**

# Sports injury

**Millions of people engage in sports on a daily basis—in schools and colleges, for recreation, and in a professional capacity. While being fit is important, every year the U.S. medical services treat more than 10 million sports-related injuries—3.5 million of which are in children under 15.**

In a society that places looks, physique, and health above everything else, sports stars like Michael Jordan, who earn millions of dollars, are seen as positive role models. Many people believe that sports keep young people off the streets and out of trouble, and teach them coordination, stamina, and how to work as part of a team. Some people claim that sports celebrities have a godlike status, and most fans want to imitate them in every way—from their perfect physiques and high earnings to their often very glamorous lifestyles. As a result, some critics claim, some sports participants push themselves or are pushed too far too fast, and may incur injury. In a best-case scenario, the injuries are minor; in the worst cases, however, injuries can result in serious medical problems.

## Types of injury

Sports injuries fall into two basic categories: acute injuries and overuse or chronic injuries.

**Acute injuries:** These are caused by a sudden trauma—from a single blow, a twist, or a fall, for example. Acute injuries include contusions (bruises that may result in swelling or bleeding in muscles and other body tissues); abrasions or scrapes (see Abrasions and Cuts); lacerations (cuts usually deep enough to require stitches; see Lacerations; Sutures); sprains (partial or complete tears of a ligament); strains (partial or complete tears of a muscle or tendon), and fractures (cracks, breaks, or shattering of bone). Sprains and strains are the most common injuries (see Sprains).

**Overuse or chronic injuries:** These occur over time and are usually the result of repetitive action. They include stress fractures (small cracks in the bone's surface often caused by overuse of the

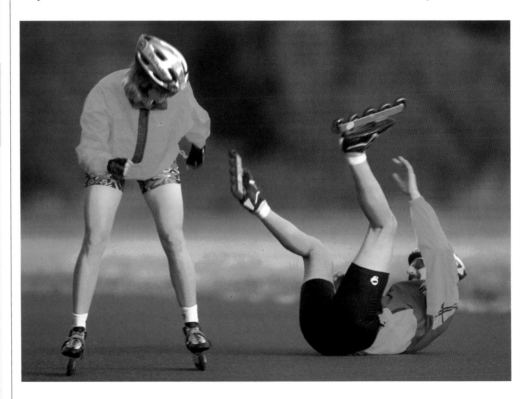

▲ *The majority of rollerblading injuries are forearm or wrist fractures, which elbow pads and wrist guards can help to prevent. Helmets and knee pads also protect against injury.*

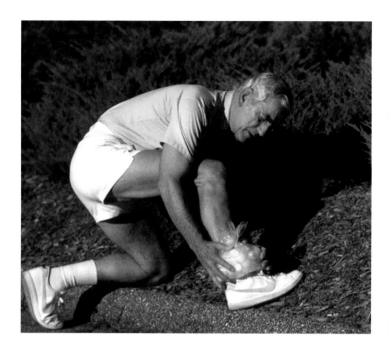

▲ *Putting an ice pack on a strain or sprain injury can help relieve pain and reduce the swelling.*

muscles used in repeated activities such as running or jumping, which then become so fatigued that they can no longer absorb the shock and transfer the stress to the bone); tendonitis (inflammation of the tendon caused by repetitive stretching); and bursitis (caused by an inflammation in the bursa sacs, located between the skin and bone in the shoulder, elbow, or knee). Overuse injuries are often not immediately visible to the eye: it is important to remember that just being unable to see an injury does not make it insignificant. Overuse injuries, if neglected, can have long-lasting effects on health.

## Treatment

Any injury should be treated as quickly and efficiently as possible. A well-equipped first aid box is essential for dealing with minor cuts and bruises. Any injury resulting in swelling, numbness, intense pain, tenderness, stiffness, or a loss of flexibility should also always be taken seriously (see Numbness; Stiffness; Swellings).

Someone who is in pain must seek the advice of a doctor, who can conduct a thorough medical examination. He or she can, if necessary, use diagnostic tools such as X rays and magnetic resonance imaging (MRI), to determine the extent of the injury (see Scans).

Once the doctor has reached a diagnosis he or she can prescribe a treatment. For a strain or sprain, for example, he or she may recommend RICE—rest, ice, compression, and elevation. Pain relief and anti-inflammatory medicines like Ibuprofen may also be prescribed (see Painkillers). Splints, casts, and surgery may also be necessary depending on the extent of the injury (see Splints).

Most doctors, especially sports doctors, will not let patients play a sport if they risk aggravating existing injuries or being further injured. They often insist that the patient stop playing the sport until the injury has healed, recommend that the patient use some kind of protection or padding like a knee brace or wrist guard, or in some cases refer the person on to a physical therapist.

The burning question on most recovering patients' lips is: when can I play again? The first point is to make sure that the existing

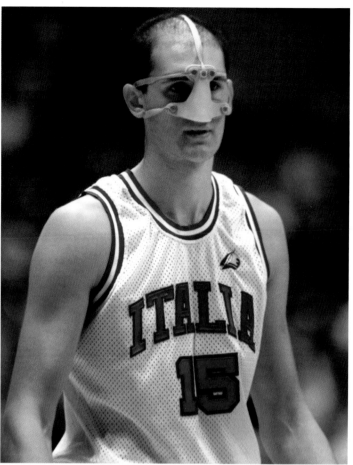

▲ *This basketball player wears a nose shield to help prevent a broken nose—a common injury in basketball.*

injury has healed properly. Staying fit while recovering is also a major concern of any sports player, especially during prolonged treatment. Low-impact activities like swimming can help maintain fitness levels, but it is important to seek medical advice before engaging in any kind of physical activity, since it may aggravate existing conditions or, even worse, create new ones (see Physical Fitness).

## Playing safely

More sports injuries occur in physical education classes and free-play sports than in organized team sports. There are, however, certain precautions that sports participants and instructors or teachers can take in order to minimize the risk of injury. The instructor or teacher should make sure the participant is in suitable physical condition to play the sport, knows and understands the rules of the sport, wears the correct protective gear (such as a helmet or body padding), and knows and has been shown how to use any relevant athletic equipment. It is also essential to make sure that the participants have warmed up properly before they begin to play and to ensure that they avoid or stop play when tired or in pain, particularly if the pain occurs on the site of an existing or old injury. If in doubt do not play; it is simply not worth the risk.

*See also:* **Bruises; Bursitis; Fractures; Ligaments; Physical therapy; Sports medicine; Tendons; Tennis elbow**

# Sports medicine

## Questions and Answers

**Should my daughter continue her sports training during her period?**

The effects of menstruation vary considerably from one woman to another. Some women are virtually incapacitated during this time; others experience little or no discomfort. Exercise can improve a woman's capacity to cope with the changes that occur during menstruation, so if your daughter is comfortable training during her period, let her continue to do so. Many women athletes find that their sporting performance varies over the menstrual cycle, usually deteriorating in the days preceding their period and picking up in midcycle, though some find that they actually perform best during their periods. Many women athletes don't menstruate at all.

**What is the value of high altitude training?**

The air at high altitudes is at a much lower pressure, so less passes to the blood than at sea level. The body compensates by increasing the concentration of hemoglobin in the blood. This allows the body to use what available oxygen there is more efficiently. This increased oxygen-carrying capacity should also help an athlete's performance when he or she returns to sea level.

**My son insists on wearing low-cut cleats when playing football. Wouldn't he be safer wearing cleats with better ankle protection?**

Ankle injuries are more common with low-cut shoes. Heavier shoes give more protection, but may cause some loss of speed and agility, and may be tiring. If your son plays in midfield, where the chance of being kicked on the ankle are higher, a heavier shoe could be used. If he plays in a rear position, in which speed and agility are more important, a lighter-weight shoe might be better.

**Virtually every sport involves some risk of injury, from the trivial to the disastrous. Sports medicine investigates the causes, determines the treatment, and recommends methods of preventing sports injuries.**

One of the most important applications of sports medicine is to study the factors that can affect fitness—including strength, speed, skill, stamina, agility, and personality—and to suggest ways in which performance can be improved through diet, training, and lifestyle (see Diet). Medical research and opinion may also make a valuable contribution to the design of sports equipment and protective clothing, and sporting authorities may turn to doctors for advice about the drugs that athletes can use without side effects. Generally, however, sports medicine is concerned with the causes, treatment, and prevention of sports injuries at all levels of participation.

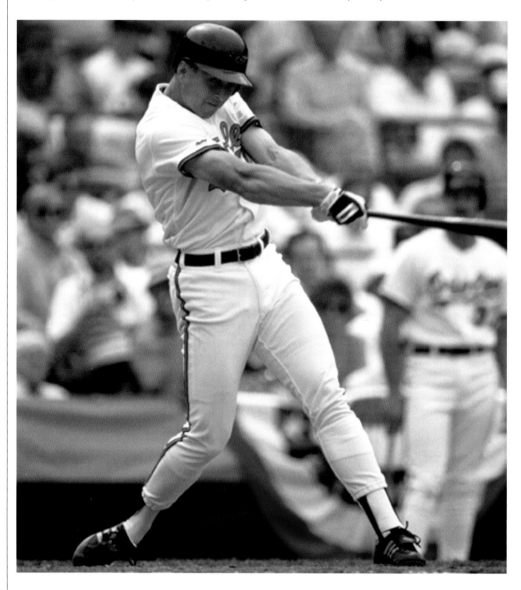

▲ *Injuries in highly competitive sports such as baseball are widespread. Protective clothing and equipment are vital to help prevent serious physical damage. Baseball players wear shin guards, padded gloves, thigh pads, and helmets to protect them from the very hard ball and from other players.*

▶ *Skiing injuries are very common.*
*Before a ski outing, special exercises that*
*condition and strengthen the main*
*muscles used in skiing are advised to help*
*prevent the most common injuries.*

## Types of sports injury

Virtually every sport involves some risk of injury, although the pattern of injury varies considerably from one sport to another. Perhaps the most hazardous sports are those involving high speed, such as motor racing and skiing; or those that involve special environmental hazards, such as scuba diving and mountaineering.

Body-contact sports, such as football, basketball, and boxing, can also pose significant dangers. In football, for example, there is the chance of an injury to virtually any part of the legs, as well as the head and collarbone, as a result of the collisions that are so commonplace. In basketball, risks include breaking an arm or leg, or being injured in a heavy tackle. Continuous heavy blows to the head in boxing may cause serious lasting damage to the brain as it is knocked around inside the skull (see Brain Damage and Disease). Cut eyes, cut mouth, cauliflower ears, broken nose, and damaged hands are also common injuries in contact sports (see Hand; Nose).

In noncontact sports, physical danger may come from the equipment used. Being hit on the head by a baseball and being spiked by a fellow athlete's track shoes are common examples. More often, injury is self-inflicted or it follows the overuse of some part of the body. Examples are strained elbows and damaged knee joints of tennis

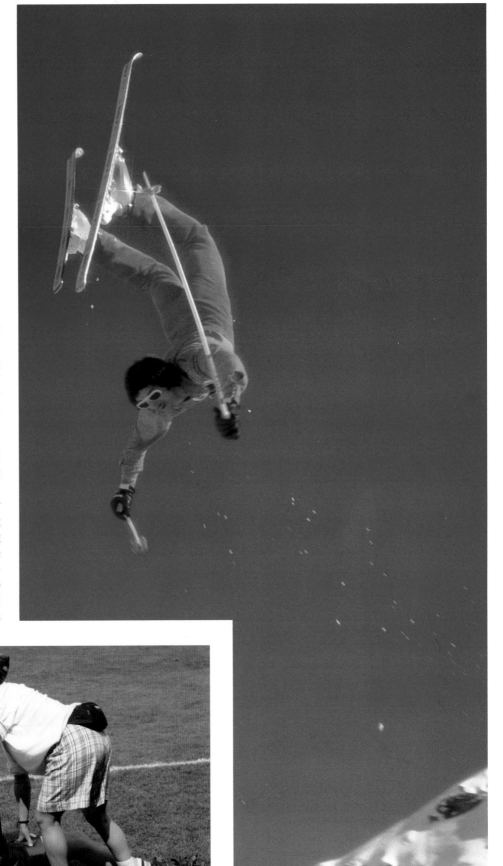

◀ *A football coach helps an injured player.*

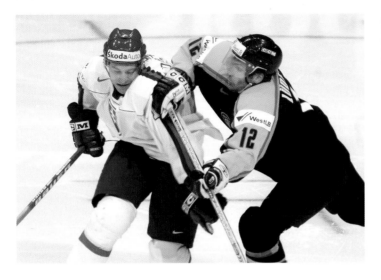

▲ *The bone-crushing sport of ice hockey makes extensive protective gear essential.*

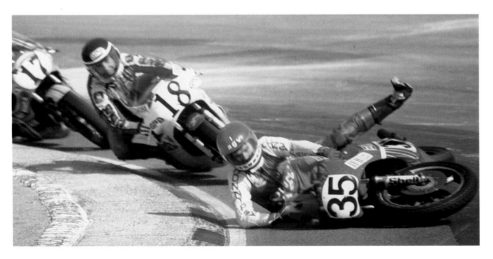

▲ *A show jumper falls from his mount. Riding helmets are essential safety gear, since falls often result in head injuries.*

players (see Elbow; Knee), pulled muscles of sprinters or throwers who have not warmed up properly before a competition, and stress fractures that sometimes affect long-distance runners in training.

## Fractures

Sports fractures may occur as the result of a direct blow, and common types of fractures include the broken legs of footballers and skiers, broken collarbones among many ballplayers, and broken finger bones, arms, and ribs in baseball players (see Ribs). Small finger and foot bones usually heal up completely after four or five weeks (see Feet), but leg fractures may require immobilization for a much longer period.

Stress fractures are overuse injuries caused by repetitive loading of a bone during training or playing. Athletes who train over very long distances each week are the most prone to this type of injury, particularly if they run mainly on roads or other hard surfaces and wear shoes without sufficient cushioned support. The bones most commonly affected are those in the middle part of the foot and the lower leg bones. Symptoms usually begin with pain in the affected area that occurs regularly during training and increases in severity

▼ *Thrills and spills of speed and power: racetrack driving is made safer by the use of helmets and leather suits.*

with each training session. At this point, the fracture may consist of a crack or a weakness in the bone structure. If the athlete rests from the activity for around four to six weeks, the injury will gradually start to heal, but to continue training in defiance of the pain could cause the bone to shatter suddenly with much more serious consequences (see Bones).

## Muscle and tendon injuries

Muscle injuries are very common in sports and usually involve a rupture of some of the muscle's fibers, variously described as a pull, a tear, or a strain. The thigh and calf muscles are the most commonly injured among footballers and the hamstrings at the back of the thigh among sprinters (see Muscles).

The usual cause of muscle strain is an excessive demand made on the muscle before it has been warmed up properly. Cold muscles contract in a jerky fashion, which can produce too great a load on some of the fibers. When they tear, the usual symptom is a sudden stabbing ache. Such pain may continue for a week or more, but it is a good idea to continue exercising gently during this time to speed the return to full activity.

Muscle stiffness is very common the morning after some unaccustomed effort, but it gradually disappears over a day or two. The stiffness is probably due to the combined effects of a number of very small tears in the muscle (see Stiffness).

Tendons are the fibrous cords that join muscles to bone. They can be ruptured or torn by a direct blow or by excessive strain, or they may become inflamed through overuse (see Inflammation). Tennis players, hockey players, and rowers often develop an inflammation of the tendons in the wrist due to a persistent tight grip on racket, stick, bat, or oar. A few days' rest usually relieves the condition.

## Joint ligament injuries

Joint injury may involve damage to the bone ends that make up the joint; to the cartilage

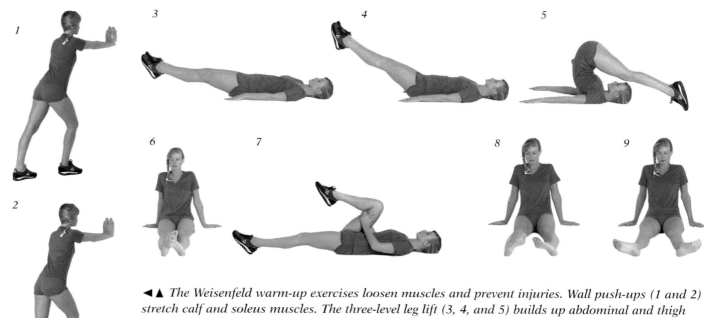

*◀▲ The Weisenfeld warm-up exercises loosen muscles and prevent injuries. Wall push-ups (1 and 2) stretch calf and soleus muscles. The three-level leg lift (3, 4, and 5) builds up abdominal and thigh muscles. The foot press exercise (6) strengthens the thigh muscles and can be used for the treatment and prevention of "runner's knee." Knee-press exercises stretch both hamstrings and lower-back muscles, preventing pulled hamstrings and lower-back pain (7). By tensing the thigh muscles, turning the feet in or out, and holding for 10 seconds (8 and 9), the thigh muscles can be strengthened.*

that coats each bone end; to the ligaments that determine the range of movement of the joint; or to a variety of other structures around and within the many different joints.

Sprains can arise when a joint is forcibly moved beyond its normal range and may involve the tearing or rupturing of a ligament; knee and ankle sprains are the most common.

Dislocations occur when one of the bone ends is completely displaced from its normal position, thus damaging the ligaments and rendering the joint either immobile or unstable. A doctor, or some other qualified person, must quickly reposition the bone before the tissues swell (see Osteopathy).

Following a sprain or a dislocation, a joint may need to be immobilized for several weeks so that the damaged ligaments can heal and regain their full strength (see Splints).

Apart from sprains and dislocations, one of the most common injuries to the knee joint is a torn cartilage, which is painful and may considerably limit any knee movement. It is quite common for damaged cartilage to require surgical removal (see Cartilage).

## Rehabilitation

Initial treatment of most sports injuries consists of measures aimed at reducing pain and swelling in the area affected, together with the resetting of fractured bones and dislocated joints, and any other first-aid measures (see Rehabilitation). Although the injured part of the body often has to be immobilized for some weeks to allow damaged tissues to heal, in many cases an early return to light exercise is encouraged to prevent muscle wasting or the formation of scar tissue that might delay full recovery (see Exercise).

A graded exercise program is worked out by doctor and physical therapist with the aim of rebuilding muscle, tendon, and bone strength or joint stability, and restoring a full range of movement (see Physical Therapy). The temptation to return to full participation in a sport before obtaining the doctor's permission should be resisted. This is likely to lead to a recurrence of the injury, followed by a further, and usually longer, spell on the sidelines.

## Avoiding injury

Most sports injuries could be avoided through a mixture of common sense, fitness training, expert supervision, and adequate preparation for the particular activity in question, which includes selecting and using the right equipment.

If a person has not had any exercise for several months, strenuous activities should be avoided until he or she has built up an appropriate level of fitness by taking part in a more moderate activity. Thorough stretching and warming up before a game will help protect the muscles and joints from injury when the game begins.

Protective clothing—such as helmets, pads, gloves, and boxes to safeguard the genitals for ice hockey and football players; shin pads for baseball players; and gum shields for boxers—should be worn wherever possible. Wearing the correct footwear is also particularly important for all types of sport. Training shoes should be comfortable and well padded with shock-absorbent material, and should have treads that provide an adequate grip on the training surface. For sports that involve rapid changes in direction, the shoe must provide adequate support to the side of the foot in order to prevent the ankle from turning.

Any persistent pain that occurs during training sessions should be dealt with by refraining from the activity for a few days. Even better, the injured person should pay a visit to the doctor. Ignoring the discomfort of a sports injury is likely to aggravate any persistent problem and also invites disaster. A person should take note and act on what his or her body is saying. (see Pain).

*See also:* **Dislocation; Fractures; Joints; Ligaments; Physical fitness; Pulled muscles; Sports injury; Sprains; Tennis elbow**

# Sprains

## Questions and Answers

**What is the best type of bandage to use in treating a sprain?**

The aim is to give the joint firm support while it heals, but it should not be completely immobilized as a fracture has to be. Some form of elasticized bandage is therefore required. An ordinary cotton bandage gives too little support, but crepe, webbing, and elastic bandages are all suitable. The bandage must be put on tightly enough to be effective, but not so tightly that it interferes with the circulation; the patient may then be in danger of getting gangrene. If the extremities (the toes in the case of a sprained ankle, and the fingers in a sprained wrist) go white, become numb, or get pins and needles, then the bandage is too tight. If this is the case, you must take it off and start again, bandaging a little more loosely.

**How are cold compresses used in the treatment of sprains?**

Very much as the name suggests. You take something like a piece of old linen, a handkerchief, a dish towel, or a roll of bandage and thoroughly soak it in cold, but not iced, water. You then wring it out so that it no longer drips, lay it on the sprained area, and bandage it in place. As soon as it begins to dry or get warm, take it off, soak it in cold water again, and repeat the process.

To have any effect on the pain and swelling of a sprain, the cold compress must be applied within the first few minutes.

**Can massage help to treat sprains?**

Perhaps. Gentle massage can be started when the immediate effects of the injury have worn off, usually on the second or third day. The area will be very tender, so only light pressure should be applied. The massage can become gradually more strenuous as the injury heals.

**A sprain is one of the most common of all injuries, and the majority of people have sprained a wrist or ankle at some time in their life. The damage almost always heals by itself, with the help of simple home treatment.**

A sprain chiefly affects the tissues around a joint, and it generally rates as more serious than a strain, but considerably less serious than a dislocation or fracture (see Dislocation; Fractures; Joints). Virtually any joint can be involved in a sprain, but some joints are far more likely to be affected than others because of their position and the strains they frequently have to bear. The ankle is particularly vulnerable because it bears much of the body's weight and is often involved in potentially hazardous activities.

## Causes

Sprains are usually the result of the sharp twisting or wrenching of a joint beyond its natural limits. If the force involved is very great there may, in addition, be dislocation or even a fracture. Most commonly, however, the ligaments are affected. These are very tough bands of fibroelastic

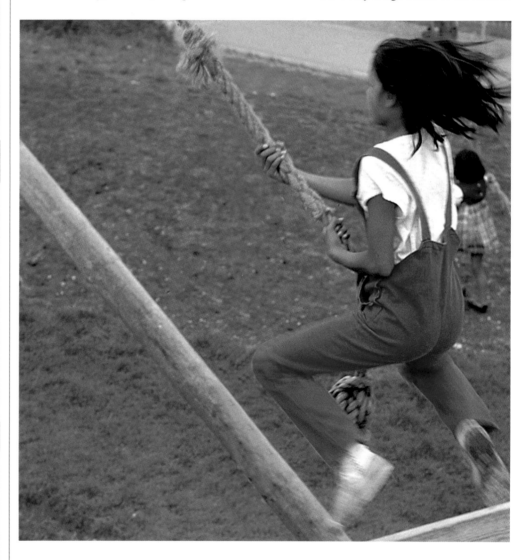

▲ *Accidents will happen when children become adventurous in their play; and a fall may result in a sprained wrist or ankle.*

tissue that hold the joint firmly in the correct position and protect it from dislocation. In trying to resist the force that is suddenly exerted on them, the ligaments may become stretched and some of the fibers may even be torn. It is rare, however, for the whole ligament to be pulled apart or ripped away from the bone. Any tendons (the thin, tough tails of muscle) may be similarly affected (see Tendons). Blood vessels in the tissues surrounding the joint are likely to be torn, causing bleeding and the bluish discoloration which is characteristic of many sprains (see Bruises).

Any accident may bring about a sprain. People may sprain their ankles when tripping on the stairs or falling off a ladder. Wrist sprains are also a common consequence of falls. The larger joints, such as the knee and hip, may be sprained in the course of a strenuous sport, and neck sprains may result from whiplash injuries when an automobile is brought to a sudden, violent halt.

## Symptoms

There are several changes in the joint that indicate it has been sprained. The most obvious is sudden, severe pain in the affected area. This comes from two sources: from the stretched or torn strands of ligament, and from distention of the surrounding tissue. This is brought about by bleeding and the secretion of fluid, which is part of the repair process.

The pain becomes dramatically worse if any attempt is made to move the joint or to make it bear any weight. As a result, there is also disability in the sense that the joint is put temporarily out of use. Any movement that is possible will be slight and of little practical value.

The swelling over the ligament usually develops quickly, and any bleeding into the underlying tissue will give it a blue or bruised appearance. As well as pain there will be tenderness. Even light pressure on the side of the joint will cause pain, but the actual site of the damage will be particularly sensitive. This is known as pinpoint tenderness, and it helps to indicate where the damage is in a swollen joint.

## Treatment and outlook

Distinguishing between a sprain and more serious damage, such as a fracture, can be very difficult, but it is essential. It should be remembered that the two types of damage are really different stages in the same process, and that both involve pain, tenderness, swelling, and loss of use of the joint. Apparent sprains, unless they are obviously very minor, must therefore be treated with great caution until a doctor's opinion has been obtained. In this way, any aggravation of a possible fracture will be avoided. An X ray may even be needed to confirm the diagnosis (see X Rays).

The treatment of sprains has undergone considerable changes over the last decades. Not all doctors, however, are in complete agreement with the newer approach, which recommends using the joint rather than resting it.

Immediate treatments, nevertheless, remain fairly standard. If a doctor is available when the sprain occurs (as may happen with a sports injury), he or she may inject the area with local anesthesia to minimize the reaction (see Local Anesthetics). A cold, but not ice, compress may be used for the same purpose, but not with such dramatic effect. The affected joint should then be firmly bandaged to limit the swelling and provide support (see Dressings and Bandages).

Heat should never be applied to a new sprain, though it may well be helpful in restoring function from the second day onward (see Heat Treatment). The patient may then start to use the joint gradually, perhaps with the help of a crutch. In most cases, however, healing will be rapid.

### Bandaging a sprained ankle

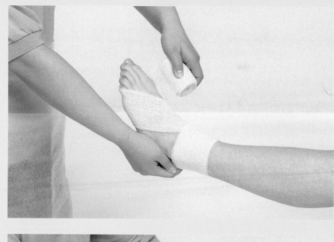

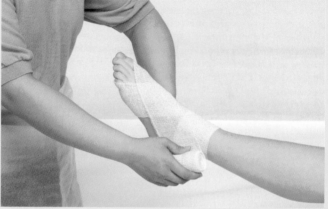

**Stand in front of the patient and position the injured foot at a right angle to the shin.**

**Use an elasticized bandage, unrolling it as you work and holding the remainder so that it faces upward.**

**Starting well up on the ankle, make a "U" shape with the bandage, taking it down under the heel and up again, so that the foot is pulled up firmly to the leg.**

**Then take the strap around the back of the lower leg and down again to form a second "U."**

**Start off with a couple of firm turns to make sure it does not slip, then apply the rest evenly and firmly. Each successive turn should cover two-thirds of the previous one.**

**Secure with a safety pin through the two outermost layers. If it works loose through wear, remove and reapply.**

*See also:* **Healing; Knee; Ligaments; Sports injury; Sports medicine; Swellings; Whiplash injury**

# Stammering and stuttering

## Questions and Answers

**My three-year-old daughter seems to be developing a stammer. Should I correct her speech or simply ignore it?**

Most children of this age go through a stage of normal nonfluency which sounds rather like a stammer. It happens because she doesn't yet have a large enough vocabulary to express herself. Don't correct her; this could make her self-conscious about her speech and she could develop a real stammer. Give her your full attention when she speaks to you and allow her time to say all she wants. Don't feel anxious, because this feeling will be communicated to her. She will then feel she is doing something wrong and also become anxious about her speech. If it persists, seek advice from a speech therapist.

**I stammer only when I feel under stress, so I haven't bothered to seek treatment for it. I have now been asked to give a speech at my son's school and don't want to let him down by refusing, but I am afraid of stammering. How can I overcome this problem?**

You can buy a machine called a masker which emits white noise into your ears when you speak; this prevents you from hearing your speech. Most people who stammer find that it keeps them fluent for such occasions as public speaking, but it is usually prescribed only as a last resort. Your local speech therapist may help you get one and teach you how to use it, but a course of speech therapy would probably be of more long-term benefit.

**Do more boys than girls stammer?**

Yes. The ratio is as high as four boys to every one girl who stammers. Girls tend to be quicker developing speech; this may be why they stammer less.

**"Stammering" and "stuttering" are both terms for the same speech difficulty—the hesitations that interrupt fluent speech. Speech therapy is used to treat speech problems.**

No one speaks with perfect fluency. It is common to hesitate and repeat phrases, but these interruptions are not usually noticed by either the speaker or the person listening. Normally the speaker is far more interested in what he or she is saying than how it is said.

People who stammer are, on the other hand, very conscious of how they speak and worry about getting the words out. Although they can speak normally under certain conditions, they cannot keep their speech fluent at all times. Stammering is more common among boys than girls, and often starts between ages three and eight.

## Normal nonfluency

Most children go through a stage when they hesitate and repeat sounds. This usually happens at about three years old, when children are eager to explain their new experiences, but don't yet have the vocabulary to express themselves. While searching for words, they fill the pause by repeating the previous phrase, previous words, or the initial sounds of words. Repetition of sounds in normal nonfluency is relaxed, and the child does not notice it unless it is drawn to his or her attention. It is important to listen when children are going through this phase without seeming to be worried about their speech. If children sense any anxiety they will start to feel they are doing something wrong and become tense about speaking. This could lead to a true stammer. Most children learn enough words to express their ideas, and this phase of nonfluency disappears. Fifty to 80 percent of childhood stammerers do not stammer as adults.

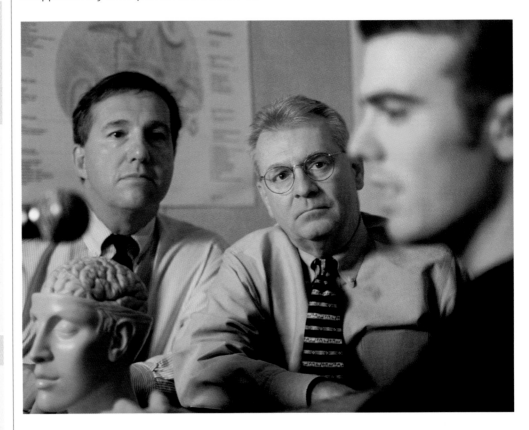

▲ *A patient is using Speecheasy, a hearing-aid device designed to assist people who stutter. Physicians are listening to him speak to assess the benefit he is getting.*

## Primary stammering

The first stage of stammering commonly appears as repetitions of the initial sounds of words. The onset is often gradual and may progress from normal nonfluency, or it may appear after an illness or trauma. Hesitations and repetitions often increase as the child becomes more anxious about certain situations. This anxiety can be exacerbated by the parents' attitude toward the child's speech problem. No one knows why some children become worried by a speech difficulty, but it is this anxiety about speaking which can result in a stammer. Often, in the early stages, the child's difficulty occurs only occasionally—such as when he or she is in a hurry, excited, or anxious to tell a story.

## Secondary stammering

There is a secondary stage of stammering that causes tension and embarrassment. Instead of repeating sounds, the stammerer cannot get sounds out at all, or once started, cannot end them. These interruptions, known as blocks and prolongations respectively, are often accompanied by eye blinks, facial tics, and limb movements (see Twitches and Tics). Blinks and tics often become part of the

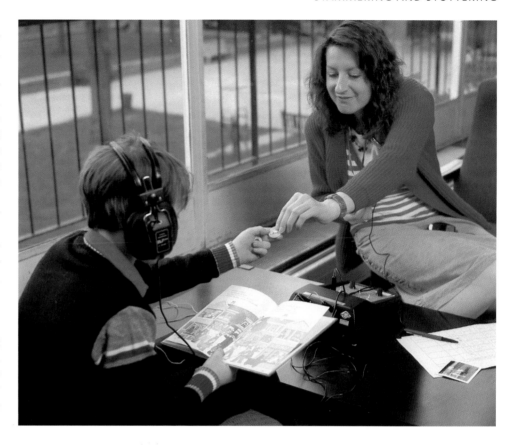

▲ *The machine slows down the speed at which a stammerer hears his or her own speech. This boy is rewarded with a token as he reads a paragraph without hesitation.*

stammer, as a chance movement sometimes seems to help the stammerer to force out a word. In reality, however, a movement has nothing to do with producing the sound, since a stammer occurs essentially because the muscles of speech are not controlled or coordinated and there is too much tension in the muscles used for breathing and sound formation.

## Points of difficulty

No particular sounds create specific problems for all stammerers, but individuals find certain sounds more difficult than others and will try to avoid them. For example, a person who thinks he or she will get stuck on "m," will say hill instead of mountain, or even use a whole phrase instead of the difficult word. The stammerer may become so skilled at avoiding words that it passes unnoticed, but ultimately it serves to reinforce his or her lack of confidence.

If a word cannot be avoided, a common trick is to add a set phrase such as "that is to say," which stammerers hope will carry them over the difficult word. On the whole, the consonants "p," "b," "t," "d," "k," and "g" create blocks, whereas sounds such as "f" and "s" result in prolongations.

The degree to which a stammer affects someone's sociability depends on his or her personality. Usually, particular situations cause anxiety and tend to be avoided. Children and adolescents fear reading in class, and adults try not to use the telephone. Often, stammerers' fear of speaking does not relate to how much they are actually stammering; when they are feeling confident they notice the stammer less, when feeling less confident, they will report the stammer as bad, even when speaking quite fluently.

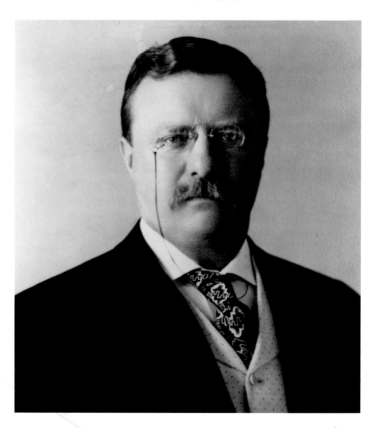

▲ *A famous stammerer, Theodore Roosevelt, proved that his speech problem did not hinder his political life.*

## Questions and Answers

**Is it possible to inherit a stammer?**

The condition can run in families but most experts do not believe that stammering is inherited. A parent may stammer yet all the children may have normal speech, or one child may stammer without influencing the speech of other children. Unconscious imitation of the speech of a parent or another child may also occur and could sound like a true stammer.

**My four-year-old son cannot say "s" properly. I correct him and now he seems to be developing a stammer. What should I do?**

It is quite normal for four-year-olds to lisp slightly. It is likely that he hasn't yet developed full control of his speech muscles, and correcting him may make him aware of a speech difficulty and he could develop a stammer. Advice should be sought from a speech therapist who will be able to organize a course of treatment to prevent a stammer.

**Will forcing a left-handed child to use his right hand cause him or her to stammer?**

This was thought to be true, but many left-handed people have learned to use their right hand successfully without any speech problems. Fear of punishment for failure to use the right hand is more likely to cause a stammer. Children are now rarely forced to use their right hand when they are naturally left-handed, so it isn't usually a problem.

**Is learning to relax useful in helping a stammerer?**

Yes, it usually does have a place in treatment. Most stammerers are fluent when they are relaxed. The problem, which a worthwhile treatment will seek to solve, is how to carry any feeling of confidence and relaxation that the stammerer has into situations which make him or her feel anxious about speaking.

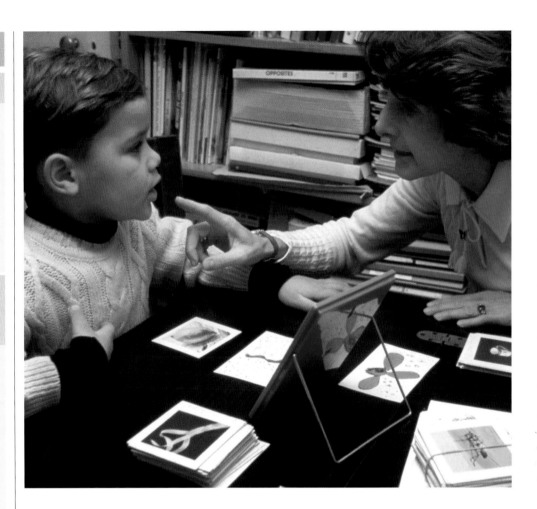

▲ *A boy who has speech and communication problems is having a speech therapy session with a speech therapist. With young children, it has been shown that the therapeutic power of play is successful in helping to develop speech.*

## Causes of stammering

No one knows what causes a stammer to develop, although many theories have been put forward. It was once thought that a left-handed person who was forced to use the right hand became a stammerer, because the normal situation, where one-half of the brain is dominant, was thereby upset, with conflicting messages being sent to the speech organs by both halves of the brain (see Speech).

Tests have shown that stammerers are as able to perform rapid and rhythmic movements as fluent speakers, and that they have no particular hormonal imbalance and are no more prone to psychological problems than other people. Most of a stammerer's personality problems are believed to be due to frustration and anxiety resulting from the stammer.

A stammer often occurs in a young child, when the control of the speech mechanism is unstable. As failure to speak fluently becomes habitual, and becomes linked with anxiety, a child learns that self-consciousness in speech is normal. Any attempt to correct the child increases his or her anxiety, so that the symptoms of stammering become part of speech, and he or she learns to speak as a stammerer.

## Assessing a stammer

Assessing the severity of a stammer in a variety of situations is crucial to devising any treatment program. Fluency must be measured by counting repetitions, prolongations, blocks, interjections, and revisions (starting a word and changing it) during reading, monologue, and conversation. The incidence of these impediments is noted (see Speech Therapy).

The attitudes of adult stammerers toward speaking are deduced through standard questionnaires and tests. If a child is young, the parents are asked to report on his or her speech at home and in school. The kinds of pressure felt by a child have to be clearly understood so that

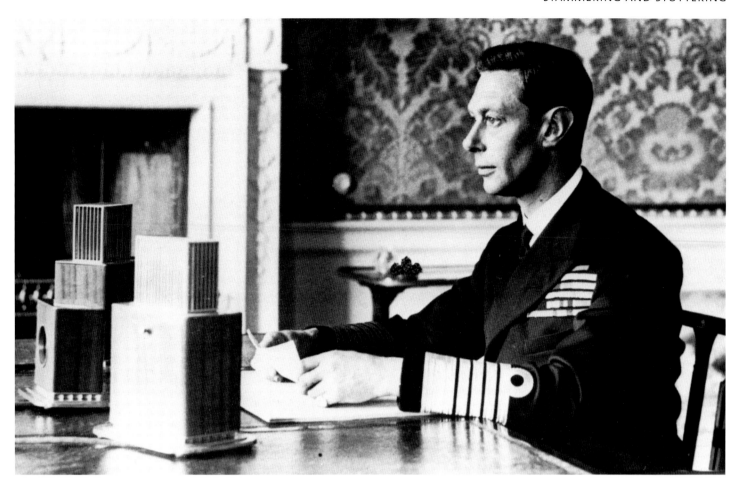

▲ *A stammer is especially disabling for public figures. The British king George VI overcame this handicap with the help of speech therapy and sheer perseverance.*

they can be reduced or alleviated by methods that are devised through the collaboration of the parents and speech therapist.

## Treatment

Any adequate treatment of stammering must treat the person as a whole. Several types of treatment work for a short time by lessening the stammerer's anxiety about speaking, because fear and the expectation of stammering are major factors in maintaining a stammering habit. However, proper speech therapy aims to teach stammerers how to control their speech, as well as helping to alter their self-image. Any therapy will be truly effective only in conjunction with the stammerer's own hard work.

The most common methods currently in use for learning fluency are slowing down the speed of speech, or prolonging the sounds of words. All stammerers can speak fluently if they allow themselves enough time to control their speech. This also enables them to speak as normal speakers do, in phrases rather than single words. As their speech control improves under the guidance of a speech therapist, they speed up their speech. Fluency programs are often used with young children: they learn to speak single words fluently, then progress to two words, three words, and so on, to continuous speech.

At the same time, the stammerer has to become accustomed to the role of a fluent speaker. Stammerers view themselves essentially as stammerers, and find it threatening to change. It is rather as if

fluent speakers were told that all the world stammers and they must do so too. As part of the treatment, therefore, the stammerer has to try out his or her newfound fluency in the real world. This is done in stages, starting with the least threatening of a series of feared speaking situations. The stammerer's therapist comes along at first, but eventually the patient is confident enough to go on these assignments alone. After several successes the patient's confidence as a fluent speaker improves.

Courses for stammerers are frequently run in groups so that they can give each other support and learn from each other's mistakes. Training in social skills should be included in the treatment because stammerers often find it difficult to approach people and talk to them in a relaxed way. The courses are usually intensive; they take place every day for two to three weeks. Most stammerers need to attend more than one course, as well as take a weekly class between courses. They can continue with classes until they feel confident enough to maintain fluency without further help.

## Outlook

As it is difficult to cure adult stammering, a stammerer may experience setbacks even after learning fluency. It is important to remember that these do not signify a permanent regression. If the person takes care to control his or her speech, fluency will return and be sufficiently maintained for the listener not to be aware of the problem. For this reason, the persistence of the stammerer is crucial in sustaining as well as achieving fluency.

See also: Anxiety; Relaxation

# Staphylococcus

**The staphylococcus is one of the most common disease-producing germs and although at one time, soon after the discovery of penicillin, it was thought that this germ had been conquered, it is now causing doctors more problems than any other bacterium.**

## Questions and Answers

**My son had a staphylococcal infection. How does a germ come to have a name like that?**

When the early bacteriologists first observed germs under a microscope, they noticed that many of them were spherical like tiny berries. The Greek word for a berry is *kokkos* so each one was called a coccus (plural cocci). Some cocci tended to form clusters resembling bunches of grapes. The Greek for a bunch of grapes is *staphyle*, so this variety of cocci were called staphylococci. When pure cultures of certain virulent staphylococci were grown on suitable media they were seen to be of a golden yellow color. The Latin for golden is *aureus*, so this species was named *Staphylococcus aureus*. *S. aureus* is a bacterium of great importance in medicine.

**What makes staphylococci stick together in clumps?**

It is what makes them prone to cause disease. *S. aureus* have on their surfaces special chemical receptors for a protein clumping factor, fibrinogen, that is present in the blood, and for proteins called fibronectins that are present on the surface membranes of body cells. The elements that cause staphylococci to stick together also cause them to stick to body cells so that they can proceed to damage or kill these cells.

**Is it true that staphylococci cause food poisoning?**

Yes. A food handler with a staphylococcal skin infection, such as a boil, especially on the hands, can contaminate the food with toxins that cause an explosive attack of illness within a few hours after the food is eaten. Infected food handlers should not have any access to food served to the public.

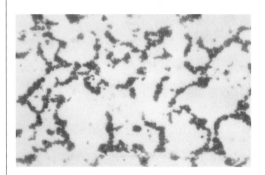

▲ Staphylococcus aureus *bacteria magnified 320 times; they cause both minor, and sometimes fatal, infections.*

Staphylococci of medical importance are spherical germs about one-thousandth of a millimeter in diameter. In the body they group into clusters like grapes. Under standard bacterial staining methods (Gram's stain) they take a dark blue color and are said to be gram-positive. The most important species is *Staphlococcus aureus* (see Bacteria).

*S. aureus* are pus-forming organisms. They cause a range of skin infections such as boils, carbuncles, abscesses, impetigo, and the dangerous scalded skin syndrome in which the layers of the skin separate from each other. They can also cause toxic shock syndrome, food poisoning, sore throat (pharyngitis), pneumonia, and an infection of the inner heart lining called endocarditis. These germs are everywhere and it is almost impossible to prevent any raw surface from becoming infected with staphylococci. They commonly infect severe burns and postoperative surgical incisions. The most dangerous aspect of staphylococci is the emergence of a strain known as MRSA that is resistant to almost all antibiotics (see Antibiotics).

## How do staphylococci cause disease?

Like many other germs, staphylococci do harm by producing a wide range of damaging factors and specific poisons (toxins) that can kill cells. Their DNA contains genes that code for adhesion factors so that they can bind on to living cells, enzymes that break down proteins, enzymes that break down the fat molecules that form cell membranes, and virulent poisons that can kill tissue cells, kill the white cells of the immune system, and break down the red cells of the blood.

*S. aureus* has shown a remarkable capacity to change so as to survive under different environmental conditions. Almost from the time antibiotics were first produced, it has developed the ability to resist destruction by one new antibiotic after another. This evolutionary process has been assisted by a tendency for doctors to prescribe antibiotics unnecessarily for trivial conditions and for patients to fail to complete full courses of antibiotic treatment.

## MRSA

After *S. aureus* became resistant to many antibiotics, a stage was reached at which infections with certain stains of it could be treated effectively only with the antibiotic methicillin. When methicillin-resistant strains began to appear, the drug was withdrawn from general use. Today, over 90 percent of hospital strains of *S. aureus* are penicillin-resistant. This is a matter of great concern, as MRSA (methicillin-resistant *Staphylococcus aureus*) are responsible for many deaths. Initially MRSA infections occurred mainly in hospitals where the environment was suitable for the rapid evolution of bacterial antibiotic resistance, but infections have now spread into the community and are becoming common there. The DNA in MRSA now codes for an enzyme that allows these strains to continue to synthesize their cell walls even if their normal penicillin-binding proteins have been inactivated by methicillin. The structure of this enzyme was recently determined, providing scientists with the hope that there may be a solution to the MRSA threat.

*See also:* **Antibiotic-resistant bacteria**

# Starch

**Starch is a complex carbohydrate that functions as a source of energy for the body. Starch is considered to be a very fattening part of our diet, but this is only the case when people consume more starch than their bodies require.**

## Questions and Answers

**Is starch more fattening than other foods?**

Only when a person eats more starch and sugar in his or her diet than any other class of food. Both fatty foods and starchy foods are easily converted to fat that is stored in the body, but only if the fat is not burned off through the appropriate amount of exercise.

**Is it possible to live without eating any starch at all in your daily diet?**

Yes, but starch is a valuable and easily obtainable source of energy, especially for active individuals. Another benefit of starch is that starchy foods are a normal source of fiber, and fiber is very important in keeping the body working well. For instance, whole wheat bread contains starch and also has a lot of fiber.

**Why can eating too much starch make you become overweight?**

The body stores a little starch in the form of glycogen, in the liver and muscles, for use when blood sugar concentrations are low. However, it is the excess glucose in the blood (the end product of the digestion of starch and sugars) that is converted to fat and deposited as fatty tissue. It is best to regard starchy foods as hidden reserves of sugar.

**In the past, people used bread and starch as poultices on their skin. What were these for and why were they commonly used?**

Poultices, or fomentations, are warm masses of pulpy material that are applied to the body to relieve pain and inflammation. Various kinds were used, and bread and starch poultices were cheap and easy to make. Starch poultices were used for the removal of scales on the skin, as well as to relieve pain.

Carbohydrates provide the body with energy, which it requires for movement, breathing, and all internal metabolic functions. People's main source of carbohydrates is starch—a complex of many molecules of sugar that must be released from it by digestive enzymes before the body can assimilate them (see Enzymes). Sugar taken in excess of energy requirements is converted to fat and deposited under the skin and elsewhere.

### Starch in the diet

People tend to eat a large amount of starch in their diets because foods rich in starch are usually cheaper and more readily available than proteins (see Protein). In itself, starch will not make a person fat; it simply provides a ready supply of glucose that the body requires for its metabolism to work.

Many weight-loss diets stress cutting down on the eating of starchy foods (see Dieting). However, a person who does enough aerobic exercise on a regular basis (see Aerobics) has little to fear from gaining weight by consuming starchy foods.

### Sources of starch

Plants manufacture carbohydrates by the process of photosynthesis, whereby they convert carbon dioxide gas from the atmosphere and water from the soil into a simple sugar, utilizing the energy from sunlight in the presence of the green pigment chlorophyll. The sugar is soluble in water and is transported to the parts of the plant that need energy for growth or repair. The excess sugar is converted into insoluble starch and stored, ready to be converted back into sugar when the plant needs it. Plants such as potatoes that have a large storage capacity therefore contain a large quantity of starch.

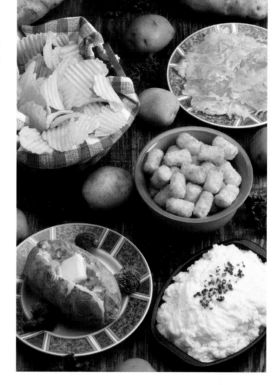

▲ *Starchy foods come in many forms, from what are known as "junk" foods, such as French fries and potato chips, to the healthy apple. Only excess starch is fattening.*

### The digestion of starch

The process of digesting starchy foods begins in the mouth. Food is first broken into manageable pieces by the teeth and mixed with the saliva produced by the salivary glands in the mouth (see Glands; Saliva). The saliva contains a starch-digesting enzyme called ptyalin, or amylase, which is capable of breaking down the starch into simpler sugars. There is, however, little time for the starch-digesting enzyme to act before the food is swallowed and passed into the stomach. In the stomach there is no digestion of carbohydrates.

When the stomach contents are passed into the duodenum, or small intestine, enzymes from the pancreas continue to break down all carbohydrates into the simple sugars like glucose that make them up. This end product of digestion is absorbed into the body, enters the hepatic portal vein, and is transported to the liver before entering the bloodstream (see Digestive System).

## STARCH METABOLISM

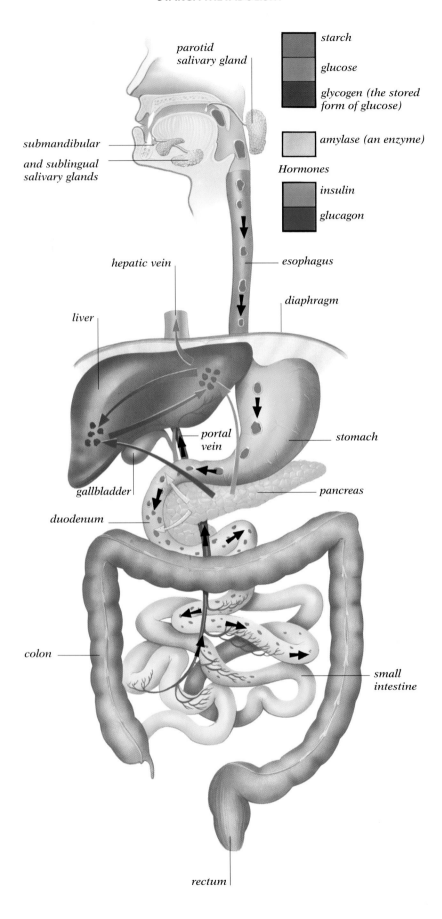

parotid salivary gland

submandibular and sublingual salivary glands

starch

glucose

glycogen (the stored form of glucose)

amylase (an enzyme)

Hormones

insulin

glucagon

esophagus

hepatic vein

diaphragm

liver

portal vein

stomach

gallbladder

pancreas

duodenum

colon

small intestine

rectum

◄ During digestion, starch is broken down into glucose by the enzyme amylase. Glucose is carried by the blood to the liver. If the level of glucose is high, insulin, a hormone from the pancreas, causes the free glucose to be converted into glycogen, which is stored in the liver. When blood glucose levels become low, the pancreas releases another hormone, glucagon, which causes the stored glycogen to be released as glucose. The body uses glucose as a fuel to provide the energy it needs for movement.

### The liver and glycogen

In the same way as plants store starch for use when sugar supplies are low, so the body also stores a small reserve of a form of starch called glycogen, or animal starch.

Glucose absorbed in the small intestine can be converted to glycogen in the liver, which usually holds about 3.5 ounces (100 g). The muscles also contain substantial quantities (see Muscles). As glucose is used up in the body to provide energy, so the equivalent amount of stored glycogen is broken down by enzymes to glucose. In this way the concentrations of glucose in the blood and body fluids can be kept within limits.

The deposition of glycogen and its reconversion to sugar are controlled by hormones, most importantly insulin from the pancreas. When people eat meals that contain a lot of starch and sugar, the amount of sugar in the blood can double within a matter of minutes. This rapid increase causes the pancreas to pour out insulin, which acts on the muscles and the liver and instructs them to withdraw sugar from the blood before it is lost in the urine, and to store it as the starch glycogen. However, the muscles and liver can store only a limited amount of starch; the excess is converted to fat and laid down in fatty tissue. Weight for weight, fats can store almost three times as much energy as starch. Obesity is the result of excess intake over energy expenditure (see Obesity).

Epinephrine and thyroid hormones are also related to glycogen breakdown and storage. These hormones accelerate the conversion of glycogen to glucose and tend to act when the body is active (see Hormones; Thyroid).

See also: Diet; Digestive system; Fats; Glucose; Liver and liver diseases; Metabolism; Sugars; Weight

# Stem cell

## Questions and Answers

**Is it true that stem cells can cure a whole range of human diseases?**

A scientist would say that careful stem cell research on mice and other animals has shown that stem cells injected into damaged tissue of all kinds can lead to a regeneration of new tissue cells of the specific type that was damaged. The potential therapeutic value of such a discovery is considerable.

**I hear that stem cells can be obtained from adults. If this is true, why is there so much argument about the use of stem cells from embryos or fetuses?**

It is true that there are plenty of stem cells in adults. These, however, do not normally give rise to any kind of body cell, as is the case with embryonic stem cells. It seems that adult stem cells normally produce only cells of the type required in their own particular location. Liver stem cells differentiate into liver cells, nervous system stem cells produce nerve tissue, muscle stem cells produce muscle cells, and so on. Embryonic stem cells can, however, produce any kind of body cell.

**Is it true that stem cells from one location in the adult body can produce different kinds of cells if transplanted elsewhere?**

There have been many reports of adult bone marrow stem cells producing muscle, heart muscle, liver, brain, and artery lining cells after transplantation. Many of these reports, however, have been found to be unduly optimistic. For instance, the tagged transplanted cells often appeared to have fused with local cells so as to give the impression that they were forming new cells of the desired type. The experts are still discussing the issue.

**The use of human stem cells in medicine is currently one of the most promising and potentially far-reaching areas of medical research and seems likely to lead to a revolution in medical science. There are, however, serious ethical problems associated with this work.**

A human egg (ovum) that has been fertilized by a spermatozoon is, briefly, a single cell. From that single cell come all the billions of cells that make up a human body. Such a cell is said to be "totipotential." This means that it is capable of differentiating into any of many different kinds of cells in the body—muscle cells, nerve cells, heart cells, kidney cells, bone cells, skin cells, blood cells, and so on. Even after the fertilized egg has divided many times to form a mass of cells, each one of these is a stem cell and each remains totipotential. An embryo, however, is not the only place where stem cells are to be found. All the blood cells produced by the bone marrow—the oxygen-carrying red cells and the whole range of white cells—derive from a stem cell. Research has shown that adult stem cells are not limited to the bone marrow; rather, they exist in many parts of the body. Production of stem cells is controlled by various hormones.

### How do stem cells produce new tissues?

Every living cell contains the whole DNA genome for the entire body of the person, animal, or plant, but at any particular location only some of the genes are required. Any cell will, typically, use only a fraction of all the genes in its DNA. If, for instance, muscle protein is needed, the genes

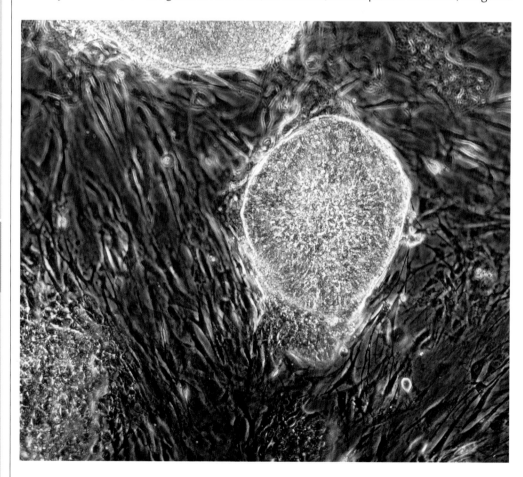

▲ *A greatly magnified stem cell seen through a microscope. All blood cells are derived from stem cells, the production of which is controlled by hormones.*

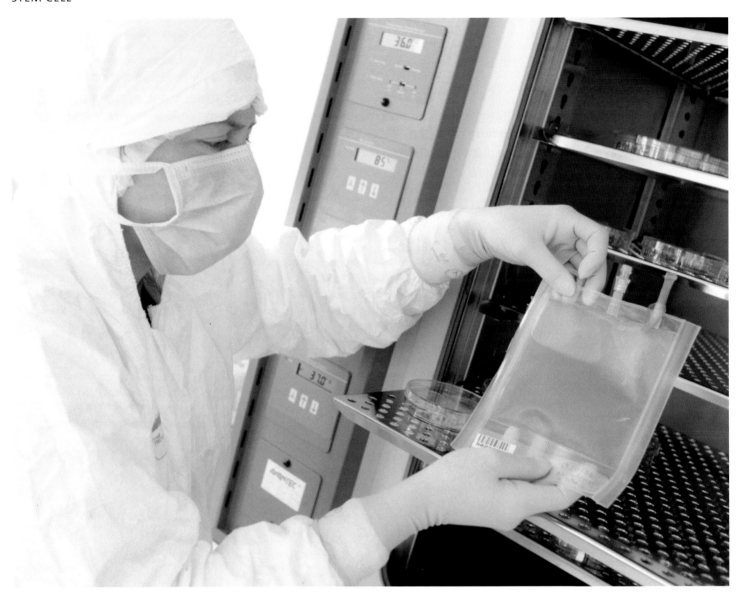

▲ *A laboratory technician is freezing a semitransparent sachet containing a blood sample taken from peripheral blood stem cell CD34.*

that code for this protein will be switched on and many other genes will be left permanently inactive. The term applied to switching on genes is "gene expression," and this occurs as a result of chemical signals from within the cell or from other cells. Gene expression can be regulated, and started or stopped, at various points in the pathway from DNA to protein.

There is now clear evidence that embryonic stem cells, if inserted into any tissue that is damaged or deficient, can continue to divide indefinitely and convert themselves into cells of the specific kind required. Thus, when a disease or disorder is caused by damage to, or shortage of, cells of a particular type, stem cell therapy should, in theory, be capable of bringing about a cure.

The list of such conditions is very long and includes heart failure, Alzheimer's disease, multiple sclerosis, liver disease, lung disease, Parkinson's disease, diabetic retinopathy, macular degeneration, and in combination with specific treatment, cancer. At present, such possibilities are, however, still in the experimental stage.

## Ethical issue

Embryonic stem cells can be obtained from fetuses that have been aborted; or embryos formed in vitro and not required for implantation; or embryos created in the laboratory as a source of stem cells. Some people believe it is justifiable to use stem cells in scientific research; many others think the use of cells from fetuses or embryos is abhorrent and ethically unacceptable (see Cloning).

## Legislation

In 2001, after review by President George W. Bush, funding was authorized for stem cell research using existing stem cell lines from human embryos before August 9. The first grants were funded by the National Institutes of Health in 2002. Certain criteria must be met before funding is granted; there must have been informed consent of the donors, the embryos must have been created for reproductive purposes and in excess of clinical need, there must be no financial inducements for the donors, and the embryos must not have been created for research purposes.

> *See also:* **Genetic diseases and disorders; Genetic engineering; Medical ethics**

# Stenosis

**The word "stenosis" means a narrowing or constriction of the diameter of a bodily passage or orifice. It may have serious effects and is of widespread importance in medicine. Almost all cases of stenosis can be corrected.**

## Questions and Answers

**My mother has stenosis and I understand it has to do with her heart. How serious is stenosis, and what kind of disease is it?**

Stenosis in the heart usually refers to one of the heart valves and means that the passage for blood through the valve has become narrowed. This may cause serious secondary effects. The most common valve to be affected is the mitral valve between the upper and lower chamber on the left side. Mitral stenosis usually implies that the valve cusps have been inflamed, then partially healed together to narrow the opening. Your mother almost certainly had rheumatic fever when she was younger.

**Soon after my son was born he was diagnosed as having congenital pyloric stenosis. What exactly does that mean and why did he have to have an operation?**

In about one baby in 1,000, the muscle ring surrounding the outlet aperture of the stomach is very thick, causing outlet obstruction. The result is projectile vomiting, hunger, and body wasting. Surgery was essential to allow the food to pass into the intestine so that your baby can receive normal nourishment. The results of surgery are excellent, recovery is rapid, and complications are rare.

**The word "stenosis" interests me. How do doctors come up with a word like that?**

Like many medical terms, it is taken from classical Greek. It comes from the Greek word *stenoun*, meaning to narrow or constrict. When the term is used to refer to a specific condition it is nearly always qualified by a reference to the organ, bodily structure, or situation in which the stenosis has occurred.

Stenosis is not a disease. It simply means an abnormal narrowing (stricture) of any bodily canal, orifice, or tube. Although any passage in the body can, in theory, suffer stenosis, there are only a limited number of places at which stenosis is common.

## Mitral and aortic stenosis

The mitral and aortic valves of the heart are those most commonly affected by stenosis. Both are on the left side of the heart. The mitral valve lies between the upper and lower chambers, that is, the atrium and ventricle respectively, and the aortic valve is at the outlet of the left ventricle. In both cases the

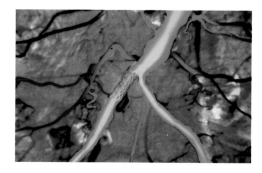

▲ *A contrast X ray, or angiogram, shows contracted stenosis of the abdominal aorta and primitive iliac arteries.*

most common cause of the narrowing is valvular inflammation and scarring occurring several decades after an attack of rheumatic fever. The condition may also, rarely, be congenital. Symptoms of mitral stenosis occur when the valve opening is reduced in area from the normal ¾ inch (5 sq cm) to about ⅓ inch (2 sq cm). The result is an abnormal rise in pressure in the left atrium and in the lungs, which drain into the left atrium. The back pressure forces the right ventricle to work harder, and its wall becomes thickened and may eventually fail to maintain the circulation (see Rheumatic Fever).

In aortic stenosis, the left ventricle becomes much enlarged and outgrows its blood supply. This leads to anginal pain on exertion and, eventually, left heart failure. In both cases valve replacement may be necessary.

## Pyloric stenosis

The pylorus is the muscle ring at the stomach outlet. When this is too thick at birth, or is narrowed by disease, food cannot pass out into the duodenum. The resulting stomach contractions cause vomiting of food eaten some time before. There is severe hunger; and unless the condition is corrected by surgery, malnutrition, emaciation, and eventually starvation will occur. Surgery to cut the muscle ring longitudinally and relieve congenital pyloric stenosis is highly successful and is now often done by endoscopy.

## Other examples of stenosis

Pulmonary stenosis is another heart valve disorder, in which the valve at the outlet of the right ventricle is narrowed. This is much less common than mitral or aortic stenosis but, like them, may be due to rheumatic fever.

Coronary artery stenosis occurs when the disease atherosclerosis forms abnormal plaques on the inside of the arteries. This narrows the arteries and limits the blood flow. As a result, the blood supply may be inadequate to support exertion, and heart pain results. This is called angina pectoris. Balloon angioplasty can effectively overcome coronary stenosis.

Laryngeal stenosis is narrowing of a part or the whole of the voice box (see Larynx and Laryngitis). This may be congenital or due to infection, injury, or disease. Anything that limits the air supply is dangerous, and in laryngeal stenosis it may be necessary, as a lifesaving procedure, to make an artificial opening into the windpipe (see Tracheostomy).

> *See also:* Stomach; Valves; Vomiting

# Sterilization

## Questions and Answers

**How easy is it to reverse a sterilization operation?**

This depends on the method used. It is possible to reverse sterilization operations in which only the fallopian tubes have been obstructed, but this is a major and expensive operation, so you will have to check if your health insurance policy covers it. Also, the operation has only a 50 percent chance of success, so it is important to realize that, if you are sterilized, it is possible that you will never have another pregnancy even if you are prepared to undergo major surgery. Therefore, before being sterilized you must be absolutely certain that you wish never to become pregnant again. This may save much heartache later.

**What are the dangers of having a sterilization procedure reversed?**

The operation itself involves a small risk, but probably the greatest risk is the possibility that, if you later conceive, the embryo will grow in a fallopian tube. This is an ectopic pregnancy. The danger is that the embryo may burst through, causing severe internal hemorrhage.

**When I recently had an abortion I asked to be sterilized at the same time, since I do not want any more children. The doctor advised me against this. Can you explain why?**

Probably the most important reason is that you are marginally more likely to develop blood clots if you are sterilized during an abortion. These clots can travel to your heart or lungs, where they are very dangerous. Also, your doctor may be worried that you could be too distressed at that time to make the correct decision on such a radical matter. This is also why doctors prefer not to sterilize a woman immediately after childbirth.

**Sterilization is an effective, once-and-for-all method of contraception, and for some women it may be a suitable step to take. However, the woman must be prepared to rule out any possibility of ever having another child.**

The term "sterilization" is now used more loosely than it was when the procedure was first put into practice. This is because, occasionally, an operation is performed to attempt to reverse a sterilization operation. Nevertheless, any woman choosing this method of contraception must be confident that she will want no more children even if her personal circumstances were to change, since it is potentially irreversible.

## Methods of sterilization

For a woman to be fertile, she must be able to release eggs from her ovaries; she must have intact fallopian tubes along which the eggs can pass to the womb; and she must have a normal womb in which the fertilized egg can embed itself and develop into a fetus and eventually a baby (see Fetus). In theory, sterilization can be achieved at any of these three sites.

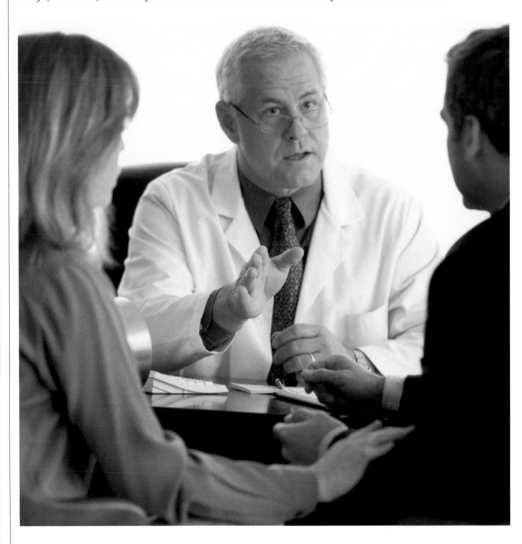

▲ *A doctor explains to a couple considering sterilization as a form of contraception exactly what the process entails. Such a consultation is essential to make sure that the couple understands the effects of the procedure, both physical and psychological.*

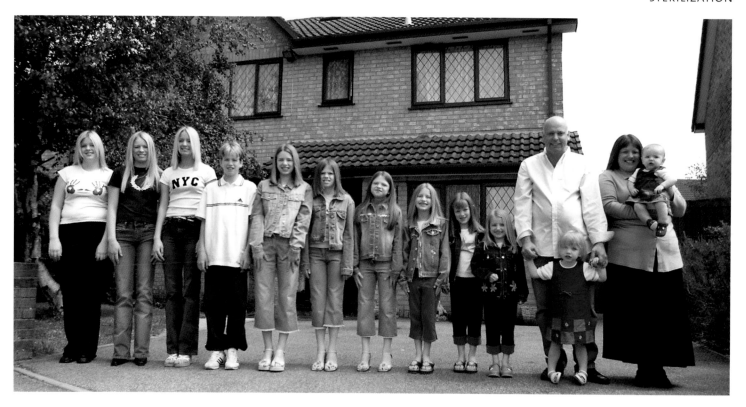

*▲ Parents Tracy and Peter Lewis are shown with their 12 children, while Tracy is pregnant with her 13th. Having produced such a large and healthy family, a couple may decide that their wishes have been amply fulfilled and seek sterilization as a means to prevent further pregnancies.*

Most sterilization procedures consist of blocking the fallopian tubes in one of a number of ways. This method is particularly popular, since it involves relatively minor surgery, though it is still a slightly more risky procedure than sterilizing a man by vasectomy. Women sterilized in this way do not have sudden menopausal symptoms (as happens when the ovaries are involved), and their periods continue, though these may be slightly heavier (see Menopause; Menstruation).

The function of the fallopian tubes may be permanently interrupted in a variety of ways. First, they may be completely removed, a method of sterilization that is unlikely to fail. Alternatively, a portion (about half an inch, roughly 1 cm) of fallopian tube may be cut away, or they may be cut through or burned—a method called diathermy. The burn is made in only two places, but the effect will travel along the tubes, thus damaging them.

In some cases, clips are placed on both tubes, or a loop of each is pulled into a tight plastic ring. All these procedures, except for total removal of the fallopian tubes, are potentially reversible, but any woman undergoing one of these operations should assume that it will make her permanently sterile. These procedures are probably the methods most often used, and seldom have any complications.

However, between one and four women in every thousand who have this type of surgery will subsequently become pregnant (see Pregnancy). This is probably because the tubes get unblocked. Another rare problem is that a fertilized egg can be trapped in one of the fallopian tubes, where it grows until it ruptures the tube and passes into the abdominal cavity. This potentially extremely dangerous condition is called an ectopic pregnancy, and is treated by surgically removing the affected tube (see Ectopic Pregnancy). These problems are nevertheless uncommon, and many women are very happy with this type of sterilization.

There are other methods which are not often used, as they are less satisfactory. It is possible, for example, to sterilize a woman by removing or damaging her ovaries, but she will then rapidly develop menopausal symptoms such as hot flashes. This method is usually contemplated only if the ovaries are already damaged or diseased.

Women and doctors seldom consider hysterectomy (the removal of the uterus) as a form of contraception because it involves major surgery. It may be a sensible choice if the woman has gynecologic problems such as large fibroids or heavy periods, both of which may be effectively cured by hysterectomy (see Fibroids).

## Advantages and disadvantages

When a woman decides to be sterilized she is making a major irreversible decision about her life that can yield many benefits. She will not have to make regular visits to the family planning clinic, and she will not have to worry about the side effects that she might otherwise have suffered with another form of contraception. She may even find that she enjoys her sex life more because she is free from the fear of an unwanted pregnancy.

However, there is always the possibility that a woman may at a later date want more children, for example if she were to form a new relationship, or if any of her children should die.

Doctors also worry about sterilizing women who are unmarried, have no children, or are very young, especially since there are successful reversible forms of contraception on the market that may suit them better (see Contraception). Of course, in every case the decision to sterilize a woman will depend ultimately on the individual herself and her doctor. For this reason it is extremely important for any woman contemplating sterilization to weigh the

## Questions and Answers

**If my sterilization failed, how would I know if I were pregnant?**

You would have the same signs of pregnancy as you would have had before you were sterilized. For example, you would miss a period, your breasts might feel tender, and you may also feel nauseated. If you feel pregnant and have a sharp pain on one or other side of your lower abdomen, you should see a doctor immediately, since there is a chance that the pregnancy is in one of the fallopian tubes (an ectopic pregnancy). This condition needs urgent treatment.

**Will I still go through menopause now that I have been sterilized?**

Menopause occurs when your ovaries can no longer release eggs. Most sterilization operations are performed on the fallopian tubes; thus the ovaries are unaffected and continue to function normally. The eggs will simply pass into the abdominal cavity, instead of into the womb. The ovaries will stop releasing eggs and ovarian hormones at menopause, so that you will have the normal menopausal symptoms.

**Is sterilization ever performed on women who have not had any children?**

This depends on whether or not the doctor consulted believes that the woman's request is reasonable. The doctor would probably consider it more reasonable if she suffered from some major physical illness that would make a pregnancy unwise, or if she carried some hereditary defect or disease.

**Will I be less feminine or put on weight if I am sterilized?**

Provided you are not sterilized by having your ovaries removed (which is very unlikely), you will have all the normal female hormones in your blood. Therefore, you should feel just as you did before, and you are unlikely to gain any weight.

### STERILIZATION BY CUTTING THE FALLOPIAN TUBES

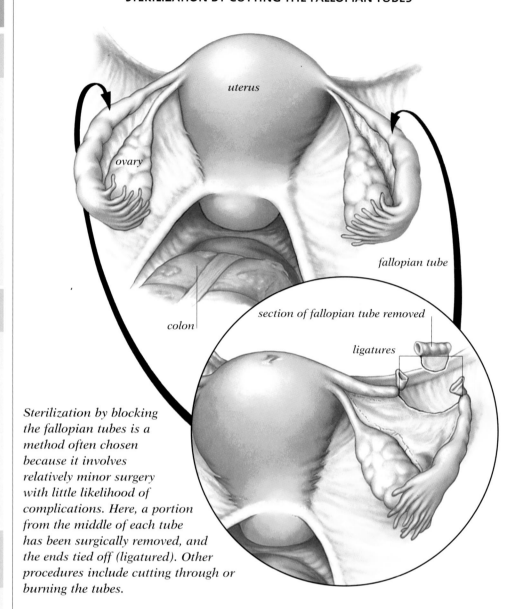

*uterus*

*ovary*

*fallopian tube*

*colon*

*section of fallopian tube removed*

*ligatures*

*Sterilization by blocking the fallopian tubes is a method often chosen because it involves relatively minor surgery with little likelihood of complications. Here, a portion from the middle of each tube has been surgically removed, and the ends tied off (ligatured). Other procedures include cutting through or burning the tubes.*

advantages and disadvantages as rationally and as carefully as possible. If a woman has any worries or questions, her physician may be able to set her mind at rest. Moreover, although the decision rests ultimately with her, she should also discuss her thoughts and feelings with her husband or partner.

### Why choose sterilization?

There seem to be three important times in a woman's life when she may consider sterilization as a form of contraception. The first may be when she is having an abortion. Although her decision is often completely rational, many doctors prefer not to sterilize a woman at the same time as an abortion is performed. There are two main reasons for this. First, she runs a greater risk of developing blood clots in her leg and pelvic veins during the operation. This is because she still has in her blood the altered levels of clotting factors that are associated with pregnancy. Second, many women may make the wrong decision at a time when they are undergoing severe emotional turmoil (see Abortion).

Similar arguments apply against sterilizing a woman immediately after having a baby, as well as the further argument that it is sensible to be certain that the new baby will thrive. Often, however, women and doctors feel that the convenience of the mother's being sterilized while still in the hospital with the baby outweighs the disadvantages. Women also choose sterilization

## Sterilization procedures

| SITE OF STERILIZATION | PROCEDURE | SURGICAL METHOD USED | GENERAL REMARKS |
|---|---|---|---|
| Fallopian tubes | Removal of both fallopian tubes. Removal of midportion of both tubes. Cutting or burning of both tubes. Placing clips on both tubes. Pulling a loop of each tube through a tight plastic ring. | Use of the laparoscope or incision through vaginal or lower abdominal wall. Incision through vaginal or lower abdominal wall. | Very unlikely to fail as a form of sterilization. Probably the most common methods used since they are relatively minor operations with a low incidence of complications. |
| Uterus | Removal of uterus (hysterectomy). | Incision in the lower abdomen. Removal through the vagina. | A method used if a woman has completed her family and has other gynecologic problems such as heavy periods or large fibroids. This method used if the woman has completed her family and has a vaginal prolapse. |
| Ovaries | Removal of both ovaries. | Transverse incision in the abdominal wall just above the pubic hair line. | Usually used only if the ovaries are diseased since this method precipitates menopause. |
| | Radiation of both ovaries. | No surgery required. | Only used if a woman is very obese and requires sterilization—she will readily become menopausal. |

as they approach middle age rather than continuing to take the Pill (see Oral Contraceptives).

### Arranging to be sterilized

Women can arrange to be sterilized by asking their gynecologist. Many gynecologists prefer to interview the woman together with her partner to be certain that they both understand exactly what the surgery entails, and the disadvantages as well as the advantages of this form of contraception. If the gynecologist is convinced that sterilization is appropriate, given all the circumstances of a case, he or she will arrange a convenient date for the surgery to be performed.

It is important that the couple continue to take contraceptive precautions until the surgery has taken place, since it is possible for a pregnancy to continue normally if conception took place just before the surgery (see Conception).

### Surgery

An instrument called a laparoscope is most commonly used in sterilization. The laparoscope is a fine rod which allows a clear view of the fallopian tubes, and along which the necessary instruments can be passed to perform the operation. Laparoscopic sterilization is occasionally done while the woman is conscious, but of course the area where the laparoscope is to be inserted is first made completely numb so that the operation is almost painless.

The majority of sterilizations are, however, performed under general anesthesia (see Anesthetics), and the woman is allowed to go home the next day. The scar will be tender for several days, and most women prefer to rest as much as possible during this time, though this, of course, is difficult if a woman has a large family.

Unlike male sterilization, female sterilization is effective immediately, so that a couple need not use any other form of contraception after the procedure.

Most women wait a week or so after being sterilized before having sexual intercourse so that their scars will have time to heal. If the woman has been sterilized by hysterectomy, her scars will take even longer to heal, and she should wait a month or even six weeks before attempting intercourse (see Healing; Intercourse).

### Outlook

Stories abound about the disastrous consequences for a woman who has her fallopian tubes blocked off. Most of these are completely untrue. The woman will not look different, become less feminine, or lose interest in sex. She will probably enjoy it more, since she no longer has to worry about the possibility of pregnancy. The surgery will not make her put on weight; she will still have periods and go through menopause in exactly the same way as if she had not been sterilized.

Most surgeons performing a sterilization are well aware that a woman does not want an unsightly scar—and in most cases the scar will eventually be hidden at the umbilicus or by her pubic hair as it regrows (see Scars).

### Screening

It is important for every woman to continue having routine Pap smears after sterilization, as she will still need to be screened against the possibility of developing cancer of the cervix.

*See also:* Cancer; Cervix and cervical smears; Gynecology; Hysterectomy; Laparoscopy; Ovaries; Pap smear; Screening; Tubal ligation; Uterus; Vasectomy

# Steroids

**Treatment with steroid drugs is one of medicine's most powerful weapons. Although they can be lifesaving, however, they can also have serious and unpleasant side effects.**

## Questions and Answers

**My doctor wants to reduce the dosage of my steroids, although they make my asthma better. Why now, when I am feeling better?**

Asthma is primarily an inflammatory disorder and steroids by inhalation are usually the most effective treatment. Adequate dosage can be achieved in most cases without risk of general (systemic) effects, but in some cases, higher dosage, and even steroids by mouth, may be necessary. In such cases, it is appropriate to reduce the dosage when a satisfactory clinical response has been achieved.

**I have Addison's disease, and have been given steroids. Will I get all sorts of side effects?**

No, this is one situation where giving the drugs is free of side effects. Addison's disease results from the failure of the adrenal glands to produce an adequate amount of steroids. The missing natural hormones are replaced by drugs. Replacement treatment does not raise the level of steroids in the body above normal, so there is no risk of side effects.

**If I need steroids, would they be in tablet form?**

Steroids can be given in many different forms; this depends on what condition the steroids are treating. If the aim is to control the effects of some aspect of the immune system, the steroids are usually given by mouth. More localized inflammation can be treated differently. Skin creams, ointments, enemas, and inhalers are all examples of how steroid treatment is applied to a specific area for a specific purpose. There are also injectable steroids, and these can be given in large doses to prevent conditions such as shock. Steroid treatment is often used in this way in emergencies.

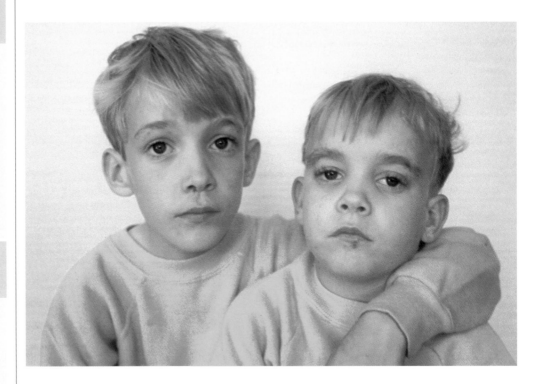

▲ *After receiving a kidney from his twin brother, Darryl (right) was given high doses of steroid drugs to suppress the body's rejection of the new organ.*

Steroids are produced naturally in the body by the adrenal glands, and these hormones are a normal and essential part of the body's endocrine system (see Adrenal Glands). The drugs that are referred to as steroids are either exactly the same as the body's naturally occurring steroids—that is, either cortisone or hydrocortisone—or else they are very closely related in both their chemical structure and their function.

Steroid drug treatment is widely used to fight both inflammation and disease, and to reduce the activity of the body's own defense system. The disadvantage of the treatment is that it can have serious side effects. Consequently, steroid treatment must be a skillful balancing act.

### The use of steroid drugs

One of the natural effects of steroid activity is to control excessive inflammation. When the body's defense system responds to infection, some of the cells that take part in attacking the infection have their activity suppressed by steroid treatment, so that their response is not vigorous enough to damage the body. This action is of interest with regard to allergy diseases, and steroids are widely used in controlling the symptoms of these allergies (see Allergies). For example, in the case of asthma, part of the allergic reaction to pollen may include severe obstruction to breathing, mainly from inflammatory swelling of the air tube linings. This response can be considerably reduced by steroid treatment. It is also possible to reduce the strength of any side effects by giving the steroids in a locally active form, such as in an inhaler.

Steroid drugs are also widely used against a group of diseases in which the body's immune system turns against itself. These include a generalized inflammatory disease known as systemic lupus erythematosus, and a similar disease, rheumatoid arthritis. There is no doubt that in the short term steroids can do much to alleviate the symptoms of these diseases. However, in the case of rheumatoid arthritis, if the treatment is used over a long period of time, the side effects will outweigh the benefits. Consequently, in treating rheumatoid arthritis it is more usually used as a short-term treatment (see Lupus; Rheumatoid Arthritis).

There are many other unusual and ill-explained inflammatory diseases that respond rapidly to steroids.

A good example is a condition called temporal arteritis, in which the walls of the arteries become inflamed for no obvious reason. This condition affects elderly people and is common in the arteries in the head, causing headaches and even blindness. Once the diagnosis is made, it improves within 24 hours of being treated with steroids.

Steroids are also the basis of the treatment of organ rejection after transplantation. The patient may be given high doses for some time to suppress the body's natural response of rejecting foreign tissue. Various tumors respond well to steroids, as well as joint inflammations such as water on the knee and tennis elbow.

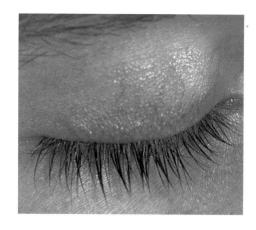

▲ *One of the side effects of steroid drug treatment is the appearance of prominent blood vessels on the eyelids. They disappear when treatment stops.*

the lining of the gut, which can lead to ulcers. Diabetes frequently occurs, and the blood pressure is raised; sometimes there may even be severe mental disturbance.

Another effect of steroid treatment is to suppress the body's own adrenal activity so that if a therapeutic dose is suddenly withdrawn, the body cannot replace it with sufficient naturally produced steroids. The danger of this is that even during a minor illness, there will be a reduced capacity to respond to stress, which can lead to shock, a sudden collapse, and loss of blood pressure. To avoid this possibility, the dose is very carefully reduced, to give the adrenal glands time to recover their own activity.

There is no doubt that steroids save many lives, and prevent even more unpleasant symptoms; however, anything but the smallest of doses can result in some side effects. Doctors attempt to keep doses as low as possible, and prescribe steroid drugs only when there is no suitable alternative available. People on long-term steroids must carry a medical identification product such as a card or bracelet giving details of their medication.

## Side effects

The unwanted side effects of steroids occur because they are given in much higher amounts than are naturally found in the body. These side effects are very similar to the symptoms of Cushing's syndrome, a disease in which the adrenal glands become overactive and so produce excessive amounts of steroid hormones in the body.

Symptoms of prolonged steroid use include excessive weight gain, with a tendency for the fat to be found on the face and trunk; and loss of protein, leading to weakness of muscles, bones, skin, and

*This model of a steroid molecule shows the basic structure common to all steroids. The molecule is composed of oxygen, hydrogen, and carbon atoms, and these are set in a pattern of 17 carbon atoms arranged in four linked rings. The chemical composition of different steroids shows changes only in the branches off the ring.*

**STEROID STRUCTURE**

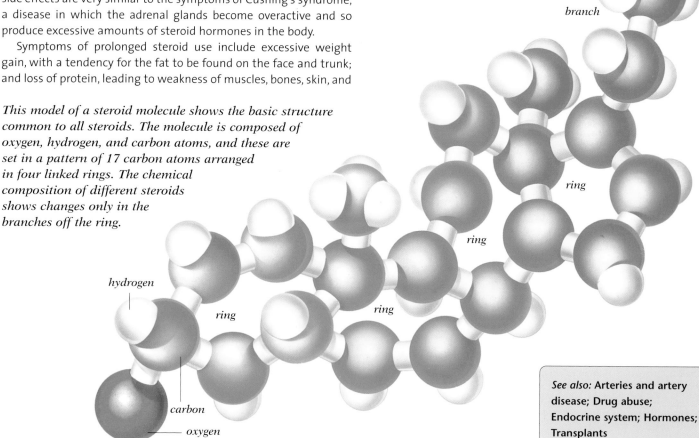

branch

ring

ring

ring

ring

hydrogen

carbon

oxygen

See also: Arteries and artery disease; Drug abuse; Endocrine system; Hormones; Transplants

# Stethoscope

**Perhaps more than any other piece of equipment, the stethoscope is a doctor's badge of office. Used most often for examinations of the heart and lungs, it is also essential for measuring blood pressure.**

**Why does a stethoscope have two pieces at the end?**

One of the pieces is called the bell; it is applied to the skin and picks up any low-frequency sounds from the heart (or any other organ). It is useful for hearing low-pitched rumbling sounds that happen as a result of heart failure or obstruction of the mitral valve. The stethoscope head rotates so that the sound channel opens into the bell or the diaphragm, which is made of plastic stretched tightly over the mouth of the bell-like end piece. It is used to hear very high-pitched blowing murmurs that can be heard when the aortic valve is diseased. Most sounds that a doctor may listen for in various organs are in the middle of the frequency range, so either the bell or the diaphragm is used.

**Why don't doctors use electronic stethoscopes; wouldn't they be able to hear better if they did?**

Electronic stethoscopes don't help much in the routine practice of medicine. The sort of sounds that doctors are listening to are quite easy to hear; the difficulty lies in their interpretation. However, one area in which electronic help is often needed is in picking up the heartbeat of a baby in the womb.

**My doctor heard a murmur in my heart and sent me to a cardiologist, who listened through a stethoscope then asked me to touch my toes 10 times. Why?**

Some heart murmurs get louder on exercise, such as the murmur from an obstructed mitral valve in the heart. The specialist was trying to make any murmur as loud as possible. However, if there was any doubt that you have such a murmur, an ultrasound test to examine the mitral valve would have decided the matter.

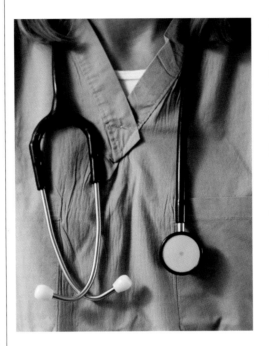

▲ A stethoscope is standard equipment for a doctor and can be used to detect problems in many organs.

▼ The modern stethoscope consists of a chest piece with a bell and diaphragm connected to the earpieces by tubing.

For centuries, doctors were unaware that the various noises produced by organs such as as the lungs and the heart are valuable in making a diagnosis. It was not until the French physician Laennec realized the potential value of these noises that the stethoscope came into being.

## Development

Laennec practiced in Paris at the end of the 18th century. At that time, a new technique of percussion had recently arrived from Vienna; the method whereby doctors tap the chest to see whether the lungs sound hollow as they should, or dull as they do if fluid is present over the lung or if the lung is becoming solid as a result of infection.

The next step after percussion was the realization that the normal sounds of breathing and of the heartbeat carried much valuable information. Initially physicians such as Laennec applied an ear directly to the patient's chest, but it is not possible to hear very well in this way.

One day Laennec saw two children playing with a long piece of wood; one was tapping one end while the other picked up the message as he listened to the other end. This

### DESIGN OF THE MODERN STETHOSCOPE

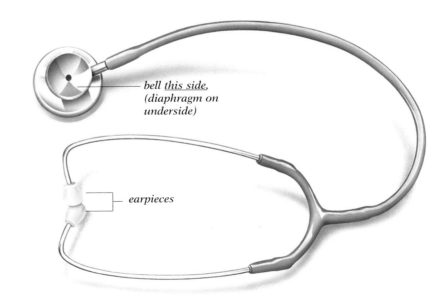

bell *this side,*
*(diaphragm on underside)*

*earpieces*

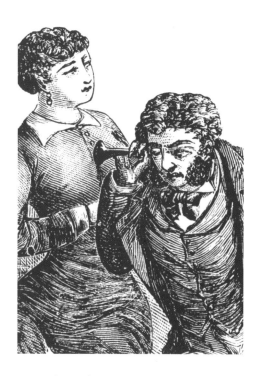

▲ *Early stethoscopes were trumpet-shaped, and the doctor listened at the smaller end. Modern obstetric stethoscopes retain this design.*

| ORGAN OR SYSTEM | USE |
|---|---|
| **Heart** | Audible murmurs, caused by disturbance of blood flow in the heart, signify valve disease. Additional sounds may indicate the presence of other heart diseases. |
| **Lungs** | Over a normal lung there is a soft rustling sound as breaths are taken. When this sound becomes harsh the underlying lung has become solid, usually as a result of infection. Additional noises, such as the wheezes that typify asthma, and fine crackling noises when fluid has collected in the alveoli, are the result of either infection or heart failure. Absence of the breath sounds suggests that there is a collection of fluid around the lung (pleural effusion). |
| **Abdomen** | Through a stethoscope, soft sounds can be heard all the time. Their absence indicates that the intestines are not working, as after an operation, for example. In contrast, very overactive sounds may indicate that the intestines are struggling hard to overcome a blockage. |
| **Uterus** | Special obstetric stethoscopes are used to detect the beating of the baby's heart during late pregnancy. |
| **Blood vessels** | The stethoscope is used over the brachial artery in the arm to establish the blood pressure. Other arteries may also be examined: a whooshing sound of blood rushing turbulently through them indicates hardening of the arteries. |
| **Thyroid gland** | Occasionally, enlargement of the thyroid gland in the neck will result in an audible rush of blood. |

**Uses of the stethoscope**

gave Laennec the idea that established the principle of the modern stethoscope. He listened to the chest of a patient through a rolled-up tube of paper and was amazed at how much he could hear. He then went on to develop a stethoscope that was trumpet-shaped. The doctor listened by putting his ear to the smaller end. The obstetric stethoscope that is used today for listening to the heart of the baby in the womb still retains much the same design.

The stethoscope then evolved to reach its current design, with a chest piece connected to the doctor's ears by a length of tubing. By the beginning of the 20th century, virtually all doctors were using such an instrument. The chest piece has varied considerably over the years, but now most stethoscopes are of the same design, with a bell and a diaphragm. The bell picks up a wide range of sounds, and it is essential for listening to the low-pitched rumbling noises produced by some diseases of the heart. The diaphragm picks up and sharpens high-pitched noises; there are various sorts of whistling and blowing murmurs from the heart that can be missed unless the diaphragm is used (see Heart Disease).

## The use of the stethoscope

Doctors find their stethoscopes of most value in diagnosing heart and lung troubles. In the heart most of the abnormal sounds are murmurs (see Murmurs of the Heart). A murmur is invariably caused by blood rushing through a constricted channel, which makes its flow confused and turbulent instead of smooth. This is what gives rise to the murmur. The doctor also listens for variations in the normal sounds of the valves as they open and close, and the possibility of extra sounds which can happen in normal young people and children, but which indicate that the heart is working under extra pressure in older people. Turbulent blood flow can also be heard in blood vessels, indicating that the vessel is slightly blocked, or that the arteries are hardening.

In the lungs there is a normal rustling noise as air moves in and out of them. When wheezing is heard, it suggests that the bronchial tubes are constricted; this may occur in asthma, whereas crackling noises indicate that there is fluid in the tiny air sacs (the alveoli). Absence of normal breath sounds may indicate a collection of fluid in the pleural space around the lungs, and alteration in the quality of the breath sounds, or in the sound when a patient speaks a test phrase such as "99," suggest that the lung is becoming solid. The stethoscope is an invaluable instrument and, when a doctor has been informed by a patient of other symptoms, a stethoscope will enable him to make a diagnosis or confirm most important diagnoses affecting the heart and the lungs (see Breathing).

## Measuring blood pressure and other uses

A stethoscope is used routinely over the brachial artery in the arm to pick up changes in sound as a blood pressure cuff is blown up. In pregnancy, the fetal heart is checked at every prenatal appointment after about 20 weeks, and it is monitored carefully throughout labor, In hospitals, the stethoscope has been largely replaced by more sophisticated electronic equipment.

*See also:* **Blood pressure**

# Stiffness

**However slight, any type of stiffness is inconvenient because it restricts movement and can be painful. Although prevention is best, knowing what to do when stiffness actually happens will minimize its effects.**

Stiffness is one of the most annoying and potentially disabling things that we can suffer from; only paralysis and severe pain interfere as much with full and free mobility.

## Common causes of stiffness

The most common and, fortunately, the least serious type of stiffness is one that we all suffer from at some time or another: muscles which we have not used strenuously for some time, or which are suddenly put to excessive or unaccustomed use, protest by becoming both stiff and sore—for example, as a result of unaccustomed gardening.

There are two distinct types of muscle stiffness. One starts during the course of exercise; the other does not develop until afterward. The first type of stiffness is due to an accumulation of a waste product called lactic acid in the muscle tissue. In the performance of its work a muscle can be compared to an automobile engine (see Muscles). It requires fuel, which is supplied by the bloodstream in the form of nutrients derived from the food we eat. This is mixed with oxygen and is then burned up to produce the energy required to make the muscle fibers contract, and produce movement. In the process, toxic waste products are produced, and unless they are

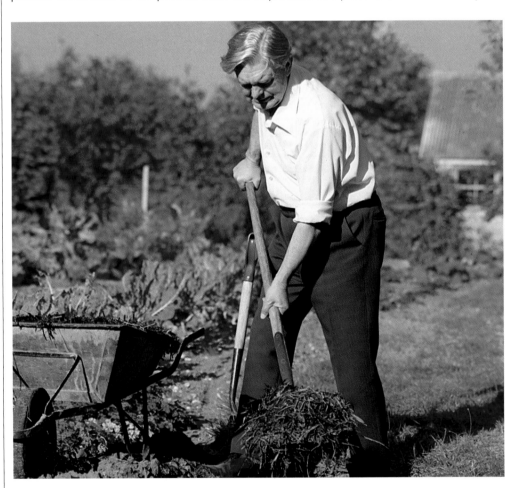

▲ *A sudden burst of strenuous work, such as digging the garden, is almost sure to result in a certain amount of stiffness if you are not used to doing it regularly.*

removed they will give rise to pain and stiffness in the muscles concerned. Usually, these waste products are removed without any problem and muscle activity is smooth and painless. Two particular circumstances, however, may cause waste products to accumulate in the muscle and cause stiffness; first, if the muscle is being used so intensely or strenuously that waste products are being produced faster than the blood can get rid of them; second, in the case of a muscle that is not usually put to such energetic use, the network of blood vessels is inadequate to permit the extra blood to be supplied that is required for both the provision of nutrients and the disposal of waste products . Stiffness that comes on after exercise is the most commonly occurring form. It is thought to result when some of the fibers of the muscle and the tissues that are intermingled with and surround the muscle become stretched, or even torn, by the unaccustomed use.

## Effects of injury

Injury to muscles or joints occurs from their being either stretched or wrenched, or as a result of direct blows causing bruising and other tissue damage. The accompanying stiffness usually disappears within a few days, when the damaged tissue has had time for repair. In some cases, however, the stiffness does not go away, and this may be due either to the part's not being allowed adequate rest or to the development of adhesions between two tissues that normally move freely across each other.

▼ *Sportsmen such as these football players need to limber up before a game; this helps to prevent muscle cramps while they are playing.*

As with any type of inflammation, injury to tissues stimulates an outflow of fluid to protect and soothe the inflamed structures. This fluid is then usually reabsorbed into the blood circulation as the inflammation subsides (see Inflammation). However, in some cases the fluid thickens to form a gluey substance instead, and this can have the effect of making neighboring tissues stick to each other. This effect is known as an adhesion. When an attempt is made to move the affected part, the adhesions make it stiff and resistant to movement and movement is painful.

Therefore, injured muscles and joints, even though being rested from their usual exertions, should regularly be put gently through their full range of movements so that adhesions do not have a chance of forming. When prolonged immobility of some part of the body is necessary—as in a fracture—this cannot be done and there is usually considerable stiffness when attempts are first made to start moving it again. This is usually in time overcome by physical therapy. Persistent adhesions, in which the stiffness does not respond to physical therapy, may require manipulation, if necessary under general anesthesia, to break them down and restore full mobility to the joint.

## Stiffness disorders

Another common cause of stiffness is inflammation of joints, a feature of all types of arthritis. It is particularly predominant in rheumatoid arthritis, a type of arthritis that primarily affects the smaller joints (see Rheumatoid Arthritis). It is often the stiffness of the finger joints, rather than pain in them, that draws attention to the condition, and stiffness may be the only symptom for several years. However, in the case of osteoarthritis, which mainly affects

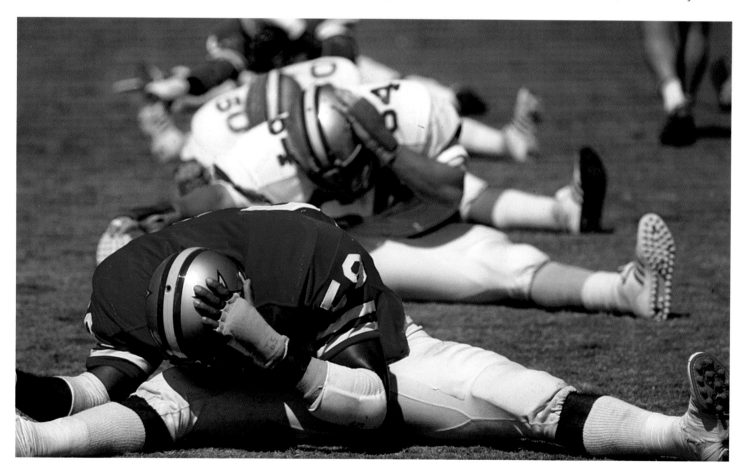

**Does massage help stiffness of the muscles. How should it be given?**

Massage seems to work in two ways. First, it breaks down any small adhesions that develop between some of the groups of tissues. Second, the physical friction of the massage stimulates the flow of blood through the part and probably enhances the repair process. A massage is best given by a trained masseur or physical therapist. In a massage, it is the friction that counts rather than oil or cream.

During a massage, gentle rubbing will not achieve much. What is required is a steady kneading movement, and pressing the balls of the thumbs well into the part concerned. It should be administered with sufficient vigor so that the massager will want to quit after 10 to 15 minutes.

**My sister developed stiffness and pain in the ankle and was given an injection right into the joint. How does this work?**

The injection used was probably one of two kinds. The first choice would be an injection of one of the synthetic cocainelike local anesthetics such as novocaine or lignocaine. When someone has a joint that is causing pain, the muscles and tendons around it tend to go into spasm to prevent it from moving and thus protect it from further damage. Spasms may become counterproductive, since they also give rise to considerable stiffness. Injecting local anesthesia into the tissues around the joint overcomes the pain, the spasm is consequently relieved, and the stiffness goes.

The second type of injection that might have been used is hydrocortisone. That would be injected directly into the joint cavity, the needle passing between the ends of the two bones. Hydrocortisone is a powerful anti-inflammatory drug, and when it is injected in this way it is able to act directly on the inflamed joint lining and thus bring about a speedy and often dramatic return to normal.

the larger joints, such as the hips and shoulders, pain usually develops first, with stiffness and disability following later (see Osteoarthritis).

Stiffness can be a problem for elderly people, both limiting their mobility and increasing their frustration. Often it is associated with particular types of arthritis and rheumatism, but more commonly there is a generally increased stiffness of all joints and muscles as part of the slowing down of physical activity that comes with aging (see Arthritis; Rheumatism).

### How the body is affected

Stiffness affects different parts of the body in particular ways. Stiffness in the neck is most commonly caused by wrenching the neck, exposure to drafts, inflamed glands, accidents, or disorders of the joints between the vertebrae of the neck (cervical spondylosis).

Stiffness of the back occurs in a variety of conditions and is often accompanied by backache (see Back and Backache). Disorders of posture, such as round shoulders (kyphosis), a sideways curve (scoliosis), or a potbelly posture (lordosis), may lead to stiffness of the back. Arthritis of any of the joints between the vertebrae will also restrict movement and give rise to stiffness. Any condition, such as lumbago or sciatica, involving considerable pain on movement of the back joints is usually accompanied by spasm or tightening of the ligaments and supporting muscles in an attempt to restrict movement, and thereby avoid pain. Stiffness usually results.

The shoulder, arm, and hand are parts of the body particularly prone to stiffness. Overuse; injuries such as sprains; arthritis and other types of inflammation; reading in bed or driving in an awkward position; exposure to drafts or damp—all can lead to stiffness in some part of the upper limbs. In older people even minor falls or twists can cause the muscles, tendons, and ligaments that surround the shoulder joint to be damaged, resulting in extreme stiffness. In the case of a frozen shoulder, there is gradually increasing stiffness and pain on movement. Nevertheless, it is important to keep the joint moving, otherwise even more severe and more persistent stiffness will result. An injection of hydrocortisone into the joint may help to reduce the inflammation and loosen the joint, but manipulation is frequently necessary.

Stiffness occurring in the elbow or in the wrists is most frequently the result of arthritis but may also be due to loose chips of bone. Stiffness of the fingers can result from a number of causes, including arthritis and accidental damage. Occasionally, there may also be inflammation of the sheath of one or more of the tendons that operate the fingers, which makes movement stiff and painful.

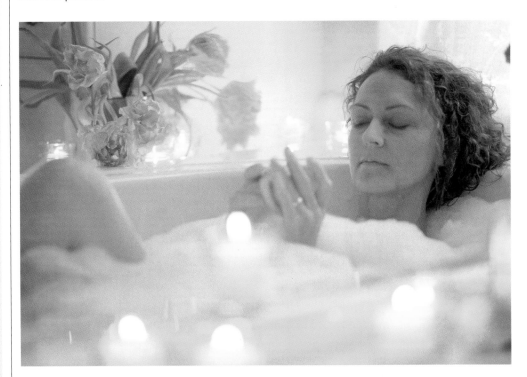

▲ *Soaking in a hot scented bath is a perfect way to relax tired muscles and ease away stiffness from the body.*

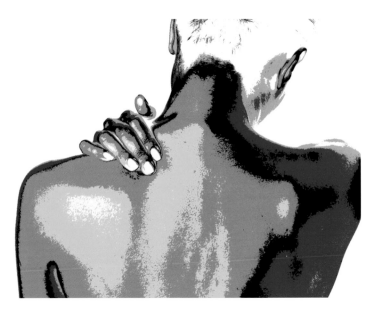

▲ *Incorrect posture can play a part in neck and shoulder stiffness. The thermal image shows a woman massaging her shoulder to relieve pain in the neck and shoulder area.*

Stiffness of the legs is mostly due to osteoarthritis, which frequently affects the hips and knees. Stiffness in the knee may be caused by a torn cartilage—though this more commonly results in episodes in which the knee becomes locked—or to the presence of loose bodies such as fragments of broken bone or torn-off cartilage. Stiffness in the ankles or the feet may be due to a previous injury, inadequately treated sprains, badly designed shoes, foot strain, or inflammation of the tendons controlling the toes. The big toe is sometimes affected by attacks of sudden stiffness and pain which make walking difficult. This is called hallux rigidus and, even though its cause is not completely understood, it should be treated promptly if permanent stiffness is to be avoided.

### Physical treatments

A variety of treatments are available for stiffness, whatever its cause and no matter which part of the body is affected. Frequently, a few days' rest from energetic use—and, in particular, from weight-bearing—is all that is needed to achieve full recovery. It is however, important that passive or assisted movements of the affected part continue on a regular basis to prevent the development of adhesions. More common forms of stiffness are likely to be helped by simple home physical therapy. Both heat and massage can bring some relief, and progressive exercises will also assist in getting the affected part back to normal (see Massage).

Obstinate cases will require additional treatment. Techniques that are available at present include physical therapy in the form of shortwave diathermy, hot packs, wax baths, hydrotherapy, and massage (see Physical Therapy).

### Drug treatments

Persistently stiff or painful joints and tendons sometimes benefit from injections of local anesthesia or of hydrocortisone, either to reduce the spasms of the surrounding tissues or to reduce inflammation. If these measures fail, or adhesions are present, it may be necessary to manipulate the joint (see Manipulation) to

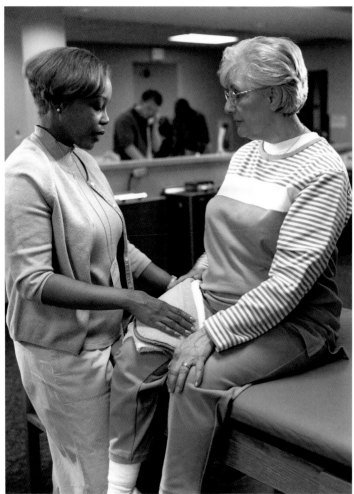

▲ *Physical therapy uses many treatments to try to overcome stiffness. In this case the physical therapist is applying a hot pack to an elderly woman to relieve the pain of stiffness.*

achieve a return to a full range of movement. If the joint is permanently damaged replacing it with an artificial joint may be possible.

Stiff joints and muscles can also be treated with other drugs. Aspirin, by virtue of its anti-inflammatory properties, will often reduce stiffness as well as pain, and is always worth trying. It should be given in soluble form or be enteric-coated, so that irritation of the stomach is avoided. There are now a large number of specifically anti-inflammatory drugs that do not contain steroids and that can achieve impressive results. If steroids themselves are used, they are given as local injections wherever possible to avoid their serious side effects (see Aspirin and Analgesics).

### Prevention

Prevention is always preferable to cure. Regular suppleness exercises throughout the middle years of life will pay dividends in avoiding premature or crippling stiffness in later years (see Physical Fitness). For people doing sporting activities, progressive training will considerably diminish the likelihood of developing disabling joint stiffness, or suffering from sports injuries.

> **See also: Physical fitness testing**

# Stillbirth

**Questions and Answers**

**My friend told me she held her stillborn baby. Isn't this morbid?**

Not at all. Many parents find it easier to grieve for a dead baby if they have seen or held him or her; and the baby becomes a person to remember.

**Is milk still produced after a woman has a stillborn baby?**

Yes, lactation does occur, but without the stimulus of a baby sucking, milk dries up quickly. Medication can help the process.

**Who can I talk to about why my baby died?**

Your obstetrician will gladly see you at the time of the death, and again about six weeks later when you have gotten over the initial shock. He or she will answer any of your questions and tell you the result of the autopsy, if there was one, on your baby.

**Why do doctors do autopsies on stillbirths? It seems heartless.**

If doctors are not sure why a baby died, it is important to find out so that they can tell the parents, and to try to prevent such a death from happening again. An autopsy may be the only way to find out the cause of death.

**Is a woman more likely to have a stillborn baby as she gets older?**

Women over 40 have an increased risk of stillbirth, but tests can be done to minimize this slight risk.

**Can alcohol or smoking cause stillbirth?**

There is a higher stillbirth rate in women who smoke and drink heavily during pregnancy.

**To lose a baby is shattering—the grief, sense of loss, and even guilt take a long time to fade. A period of mourning is necessary before the bereaved parents can come to terms with their loss and look forward to the future.**

The term "stillbirth" is used when the death of a baby occurs before it is born, but after 20 weeks or more of pregnancy. Most deaths occur while the baby is still in the uterus, before labor begins, but about 10 percent occur during labor. If a fetus dies before 28 weeks of pregnancy, the term "abortion" or "miscarriage" is used.

## Causes of stillbirth

Each year more than 26,000 women are reported to have a stillbirth, and the cause of more than half of these stillbirths is unknown. More than half of these fetal deaths are of 28 weeks or more

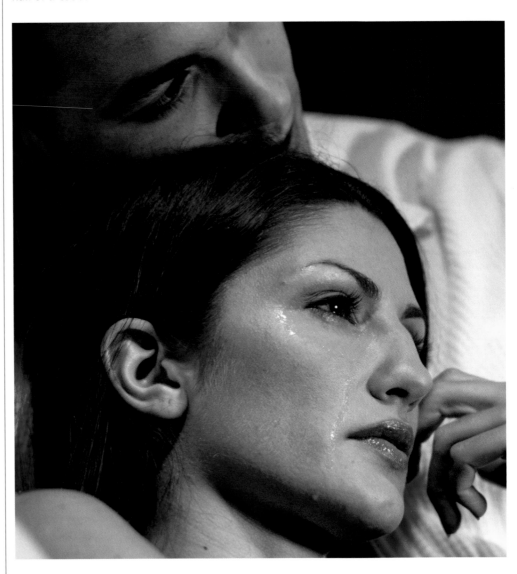

▲ *After the death of a baby there is usually a phase of shock during which the parents will need to express their grief, to cry, and to talk about their feelings. Sharing their sense of loss with each other will bring some comfort, but the time individuals take to come to terms with the experience, and to look to the future, will vary.*

gestation, and 20 percent are at full-term gestation. Although infant mortality declined by about 32 percent between 1985 and 1998, the rate of stillbirths in the same period declined by about only 14 percent. Studies have been limited because of underreporting of stillbirths; also, certification about the cause of death is sometimes lacking, there is no standardization regarding postmortem investigation and fetal autopsy rates are low, and there are few detailed geographic, population-based investigations of fetal risk factors associated with stillbirth. A body of medical evidence gives an explanation for some stillbirths. It has been suggested that some occur when there is an inadequate supply of oxygen in the blood to the baby from the mother through the umbilical cord and the placenta.

### Placental problems

One of the most common known causes of stillbirth is an abnormal separation of the afterbirth (placenta) from the inner wall of the uterus. Called placental abruption, the separation deprives the growing baby of its nutritional and oxygenated blood supply. Abruption most commonly occurs around the 35th week of pregnancy and can be diagnosed by ultrasound examination. There is often heavy bleeding in the uterus. Abruption is more common in mothers who smoke or who use cocaine (see Ultrasound).

Blood vessels in the placenta may clot; this is known as an infarction. Or, sometimes, the placenta does not seem to work very efficiently. All these conditions can predispose to a stillbirth.

Many mothers who catch rubella (see Rubella) in early pregnancy, or who have chronic kidney disease or thyroid disease, or a severe infection during pregnancy, may have a stillborn child. Some women suffer from toxemia of pregnancy; in this condition, blood pressure is high, protein is lost in the urine, and fluid is retained. With these symptoms, there is much more likelihood of having a stillborn child, and mothers must be carefully monitored during pregnancy.

### Problems during pregnancy

About 20 percent of stillbirths are caused because the baby has an abnormality—he or she may have a chromosomal disorder such as Down syndrome, or a congenital abnormality like spina bifida, or anencephaly. There may be heart or kidney abnormalities. These can be diagnosed by amniocentesis or with an ultrasound scan. Despite a successful diagnosis, a stillbirth cannot always be prevented. Women who develop preeclampsia have twice the normal risk of placental abruption.

### Rh factor

Rh incompatibility (see Rhesus Factor) used to be a major cause of stillbirth, but this condition can now be prevented by giving every Rh-negative mother an injection of anti-D gamma globulin after delivery of a Rh-positive baby, or following an abortion or stillbirth. This destroys antibodies formed during pregnancy.

### Problems during labor

A stillbirth can occur during labor. If the baby is very large relative to the size of the mother's pelvis, or is lying abnormally in the womb, or if there is more than one baby, the delivery may be difficult and the blood and oxygen supply to the baby can become obstructed. The umbilical cord can come out before the baby, or be torn, twisted in a knot, or wound around the baby's neck. The result would be to interfere with the baby's supply of oxygen from the mother.

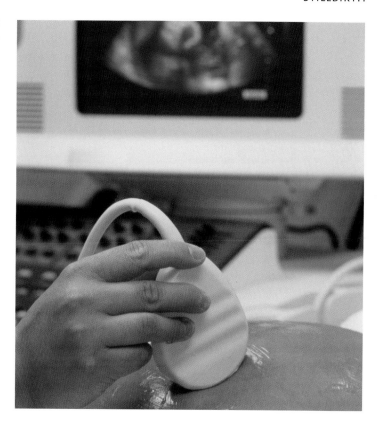

▲ *If a woman feels that her baby is not moving, the hospital will check by doing an ultrasound scan. This will show if the baby is alive and moving.*

Premature babies are much more susceptible to trauma and lack of oxygen during delivery than term babies, and hence they are at a much greater risk of being stillborn.

### Symptoms

Many women notice that their baby moves much less in the last few days before a stillbirth happens. Others will feel very jerky movements—as though the baby is trying to escape from the womb. Many women do not notice that anything has changed. Once the baby has died, no movements whatsoever will be detected by the mother. Death is confirmed if a doctor or nurse is unable to hear any fetal heartbeat, and when there have been no movements for more than 12 hours. This can be checked with an ultrasound scan or, if the baby has been dead for several days, with an X ray. If death occurs during a baby's delivery there will be no sign of life whatsoever (heartbeats, attempts to breathe, or movement) at birth.

### After the death

Once the doctor is certain that the baby is dead, he or she will tell the parents, preferably when they are together. If the fetus is still in the uterus, labor will be induced as soon as possible. Otherwise, it might take four weeks for labor to occur spontaneously; this would be extremely difficult for a woman to bear emotionally. The dead fetus can also cause the mother to bleed if it is not removed early enough. Once delivered of the fetus, the mother needs the same care as if her baby had lived, but arrangements for her to go home as soon as possible will be made with her doctor, and an appointment booked for her postnatal check.

**If the fetus dies in the womb, is it removed by a cesarean section?**

No, it is extremely rare for this to happen. Labor is usually induced by inserting a prostaglandin pessary in the vagina, near the cervix. Sometimes an oxytocin drip is also needed and the fetus is then delivered vaginally.

**When I visited my sister and her baby in the hospital, there was a woman who had had a stillborn baby. This seemed cruel. Why wasn't she put on another floor?**

Sometimes women want to face other children immediately after losing a baby; sometimes there just isn't a single room or cubicle available. It is important, too, that she should not feel totally isolated from everyone else; she can derive support and comfort from the other mothers at this very difficult time.

**My sister was told to wait until she had recovered from the death of her stillborn baby before she became pregnant again. Isn't it better to have another baby as soon as possible?**

No, it seems better for parents to learn to accept their baby's death, and this will take time. Another baby will not replace the child they have lost; it has a permanent place in the family and must be mourned properly.

**I have diabetes. Does this make me more likely to have a stillborn baby?**

If you have diabetes there is a slightly higher risk of stillbirth, but if your diabetes is controlled properly at the time of conception, and during the pregnancy, there is a much higher chance of having a normal healthy baby. See your gynecologist as soon as you start thinking about having a baby. He or she will advise you on personal care before and during your pregnancy and will undertake the necessary prenatal checkups.

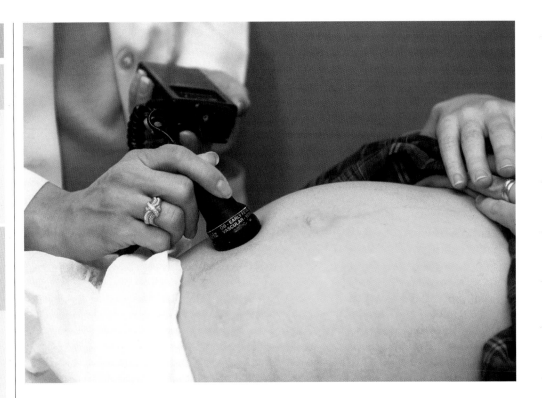

▲ *By monitoring the heartbeat of the baby in the uterus, the obstetric staff can determine whether he or she is showing any signs of distress. If the baby is being deprived of oxygen, a factor that may cause a stillbirth, a cesarean can be performed.*

### Plans to determine the causes of stillbirth

Criteria for reporting stillbirths vary from state to state; for this reason, collecting information about stillbirths has traditionally been difficult. In 2002, the National Institute of Child Health and Human Development (NICHD) awarded a grant of $3 million to fund a national research project to study stillbirth in the United States. Five research centers will spend five years collecting and analyzing data to determine the cause of stillbirth. Another aim of the project is to develop standardized research guidelines to report and investigate stillbirths.

### Grieving

Initially after the death of a baby there is a phase of shock. This can last about two months, and many parents during this time will need to express their grief, to cry, and to talk about any guilt feelings they may have. Other children in the family will also need to be comforted.

It is very common for a depressive phase to follow; some couples will search for someone, or something, to blame for the death: it may be a particular doctor, nurse, or hospital; it may be themselves. The time it takes for different individuals to adjust will obviously vary, but eventually acceptance will be reached, and with it, a willingness for normal family life to continue.

### Prevention

In nearly 40 percent of cases, the stillbirth might have been prevented if certain factors had been detected and dealt with. Good prenatal care and good obstetric care during labor are essential. The baby's growth, movement, and heart rate, as well as the mother's health, must be regularly checked. Many women still do not have adequate prenatal checks, or they start prenatal care late in their pregnancy. Sometimes, it is because they dislike the formality of, the size of, or the wait at the clinics; or there is no one to look after their other children. But it is these women who have the highest number of stillbirths (see Prenatal Care). Community hospitals may offer good prenatal care for women who do not have adequate health insurance. Any woman who suspects that her baby is not moving normally should call her obstetrician as soon as possible to prevent a stillbirth.

*See also:* Abortion; Amniocentesis

# Stimulants

## Questions and Answers

**I feel tired and run-down a lot of the time. Would a stimulant help? If so, which would be the best?**

As you can imagine, the drug company that discovers a drug that lifts people up when they are run-down is bound to make a fortune. The fact is that feeling run-down on occasion is normal. In some cases, however, the persistent feeling of being listless and run-down can be a symptom of illness or depression, and here drugs may be very valuable. Still, there is no effective and healthy pick-me-up for those of us who are just feeling a bit down from time to time.

**What is the difference between a stimulant and a tonic?**

There are various drugs that act on the nervous system, and other parts of the body, to increase the level of activity; these are the true stimulants. Tonics, which were popular in the past, are harmless compounds that were given to patients in the hope of toning them up. If tonics were effective, it was because the patient and doctor believed in their effectiveness, not because they had any direct effect on the body. This effect is known as a placebo action.

**If someone is suffering from heart failure, can a stimulant be given to make the heart work harder?**

Yes. For 200 years the treatment for heart failure depended on the stimulant activity of the drug digoxin. However, heart failure occurs because the heart muscle has been damaged so badly that it can no longer pump strongly enough. By stimulating it, you may be getting more work out of it, but you are also increasing the demand for oxygen, so overall this treatment is less effective than had been hoped for. For this reason, it is no longer the main method for treating heart failure.

**Most people use stimulant drugs more than once a day—like caffeine, the active ingredient in coffee and tea. However, there are other stimulants in use, of which some are harmful and others have specific medical uses.**

For centuries, people have been looking for some substance that would stimulate the brain, and help them overcome the vague feelings of ill health and tiredness that are part of the human condition (see Fatigue). The quest seems to be hopeless, and it is better to accept that people cannot feel 100 percent well all the time.

## Amphetamines

One group of drugs that have come nearest to fulfilling this idea of an all-around tonic is amphetamines. These drugs have an effect at most levels in the nervous system: they are able to stimulate both thought and action, while putting off the need for either sleep or food. A price has to be paid, however: if fatigue is postponed for too long, it will eventually break through, and will be more severe than before. Prolonged use can lead to a nervous, agitated state that may progress to severe psychiatric disturbance.

Amphetamines are addictive in the sense that people become unable to do without them, even though there are no serious physical withdrawal symptoms as there are with heroin. Amphetamines combined with barbiturates, which generally depress the nervous system, were once available. Some of the most common types were known as purple hearts, and these led to serious addiction problems in the 1960s. Such combinations are no longer prescribed (see Barbiturates).

Amphetamines now have only the most limited of medical uses. They are used to overcome failures of the hypothalamus, and related parts of the brain which control such functions as

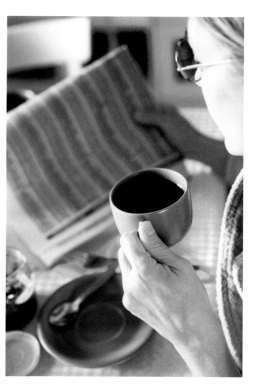

▲ *Caffeine, in the form of tea or coffee, is a stimulant that many people use in the morning to kick-start their day.*

eating and sleeping (see Appetite; Brain; Hypothalamus). Narcolepsy is a condition in which there is a frequent and irresistible desire to sleep, even in the daytime. It often results from tumors in the region of the hypothalamus, and its effects can be combated with the use of amphetamines. Oddly enough, these drugs have also been found to be useful in the treatment of overactive children.

Although doctors have become aware of the dangers of amphetamines as addictive drugs, there is no doubt that habituation to them has been growing.

## Caffeine

Western society has used caffeine for a good deal longer than amphetamines. Coffee came into widespread use in the 17th century, and caffeine has become the most socially acceptable of drugs. It poses none of the problems that are associated with excessive consumption of alcohol, and none of the health risks associated with nicotine. Alcohol and nicotine are the only other drugs to rival caffeine with regard to the amounts in which they are consumed (see Alcoholism).

Coffee is not the only substance to contain caffeine. It is also found in tea, cocoa, and cola

## EFFECTS OF STIMULANTS

## Questions and Answers

### Is coffee really a kind of stimulant?

Yes. Coffee has a nonspecific stimulating action on the brain, and this is produced by the action of caffeine, which is present in both coffee and tea. Many people find that coffee is so effective at stimulating the arousal system that they cannot drink it in the evening, since it prevents sleep.

### Is it true that the really effective tonics all have strychnine in them?

Many tonics used to have strychnine present in them in very small amounts. This gave a tonic a characteristic bitter taste. Usage probably started when it was realized that people dying of strychnine poisoning were actually suffering from overstimulation of the nervous system, with all the cells firing off at once. It was hoped that a small dose would lead to just the right amount of stimulation. However, strychnine-containing tonics are no longer available.

### I went to my doctor feeling depressed. He gave me pills, saying they would take about three weeks to work. Were these a stimulant?

No. It sounds as though your doctor found that you were depressed and gave you some tablets that reverse the chemical changes found in the brain of depressed people. These antidepressant tablets are often very effective, but they often do take three weeks to work.

### Are stimulants physically addictive?

There are many different types of stimulants, but few are addictive. The only group that causes problems are the amphetamine-like drugs, which are the most effective stimulants of brain activity and thought processes. The misuse of these drugs is widespread, but dependence is more psychological than a true physical addiction of the kind found with morphine and heroin.

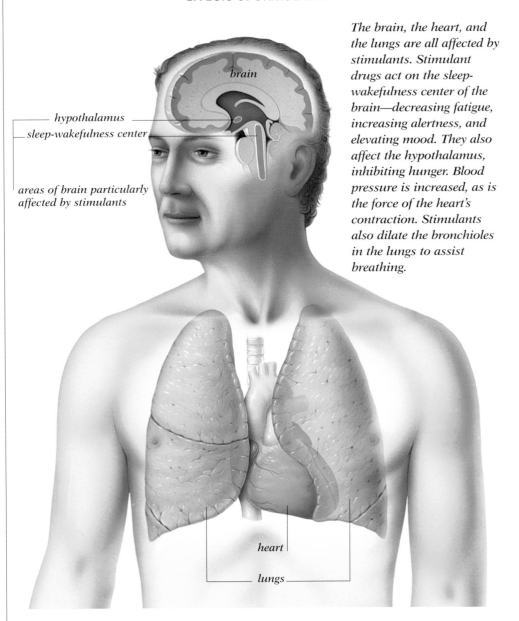

*The brain, the heart, and the lungs are all affected by stimulants. Stimulant drugs act on the sleep-wakefulness center of the brain—decreasing fatigue, increasing alertness, and elevating mood. They also affect the hypothalamus, inhibiting hunger. Blood pressure is increased, as is the force of the heart's contraction. Stimulants also dilate the bronchioles in the lungs to assist breathing.*

drinks that are made from the kola nut. All these substances also contain related compounds, for instance theobromine, and all belong to the group of xanthine derivatives.

Caffeine stimulates the central nervous system at all levels (see Nervous System), although the extent of this stimulation is less than is found with the amphetamines. Caffeine has been shown to increase ability at a variety of tasks. Overall, however, caffeine is probably incapable of improving the level of intellectual performance, although it may be able to help in maintaining a high level of functioning thought processes in circumstances in which they would otherwise be declining, as a result of tiredness or boredom.

Caffeine also effects organs outside the nervous system. Large amounts of coffee or tea have a mild diuretic effect on the kidneys (see Diuretics) and may affect the heart: the pulse rate tends to increase and some people may even get palpitations—or even panic attacks—as a result (see Anxiety). Depressed patients may abuse caffeinated drinks in order to mask their symptoms.

Caffeine is not totally without adverse effects. Drunk in large amounts, caffeine can lead to a nervous and slightly trembling state. Some degree of addiction almost certainly happens. Much more important is the fact that coffee probably contributes to many attacks of migraine. Studies have failed to show evidence that coffee is involved in causing heart attacks. However, there is a relationship between drinking more than an average amount of coffee and smoking cigarettes, and cigarettes have been proved to be a cause of heart attacks.

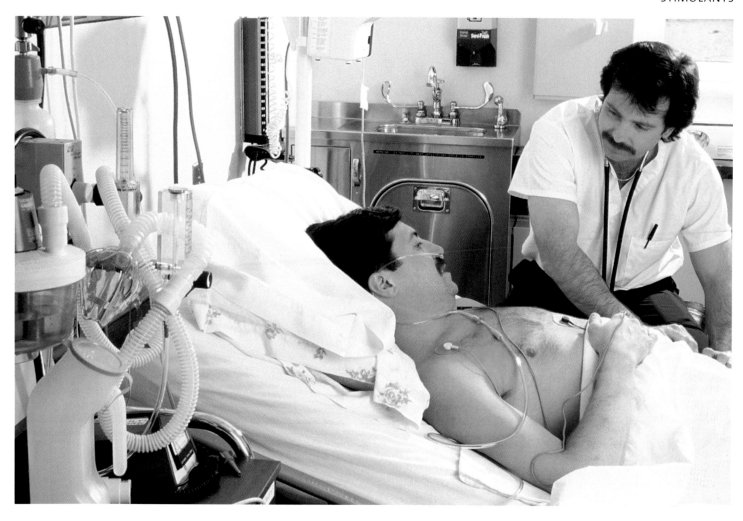

Although studies have never proved that caffeine has deleterious effects for pregnant or nursing women, most obstetricians still recommend a decreased intake of caffeine (see Pregnancy). Caffeine can, however, cause the esophageal muscle to open, allowing digestive acids to flow back into the throat.

Caffeine is closely related to another of the xanthine derivatives, a drug called aminophylline, which is one of the most useful stimulant drugs. Like caffeine, this drug works by increasing one of the messenger substances found inside the cells; this is a substance called cyclic AMP (adenosine monophosphate). This intracellular substance is responsible for turning on the various activities of many of the body's cells. Aminophylline acts more on the lungs and the heart than on the brain, like caffeine. It is very useful in dilating the bronchial tubes that become constricted and lead to an attack of asthma (see Lung and Lung Diseases), while it stimulates the heart to contract with more power. Because xanthine drugs and caffeine also magnify each other's effects, they should be used together with caution.

## Other stimulants

Epinephrine (adrenaline), the body's hormone of fight or flight, is really the most powerful of the all-around stimulants (see Adrenal Glands; Hormones). It increases the force of contraction of the heart, widens the air passages, and leads to an increase of blood flow to crucial areas like the muscles, while diverting blood from such areas as the skin and the stomach.

▲ *A patient who is having difficulty breathing may be put on a respirator, but occasionally the drug doxapram may be used to stimulate the lungs.*

Many of the drugs that doctors use are based on molecules like the epinephrine molecule. There is a whole range of stimulating drugs designed to have effects like widening the bronchial tubes in asthma, or stimulating the power of the heart's contraction if cardiac failure occurs after a heart attack or heart surgery. Another group of drugs is designed to block the effects on the heart, since overstimulation can lead to angina (pain resulting from a loss of blood supply to the heart).

Occasionally, doctors try to stimulate breathing rather than put patients on a respirator. Of the small group of drugs that do this, the most commonly used is doxapram. This drug is related in its effects to the poison strychnine, and is one of the only drugs among a group known as the analeptics that are utilized in everyday medicine. These drugs cause significant stimulation of the entire nervous system, and the smallest doses are likely to cause fits or convulsions. Doxapram will do this in a large dose, but in smaller doses it has a useful stimulating effect on the respiratory system center (the part of the brain found in the medulla that controls breathing).

See also: **Amphetamines; Depression; Heartburn; Nicotine; Psychotropic drugs**

# Stitch

**The sharp, stabbing pain of a stitch often occurs after exercise. A stitch is usually caused by a cramp in the breathing muscles, and can be temporarily debilitating.**

The term "stitch" originated as meaning any sharp, stabbing pain, such as that caused by the prick of a needle. Currently, however, a stitch is a form of cramp that produces a stabbing pain originating in the intercostal muscles or diaphragm, that is, in the front of the body around the area of the rib cage, or in the side just below the ribs.

Like other kinds of cramp, a stitch is most commonly experienced during vigorous exercise, but it can occur for no apparent reason. Although painful and temporarily debilitating, a stitch

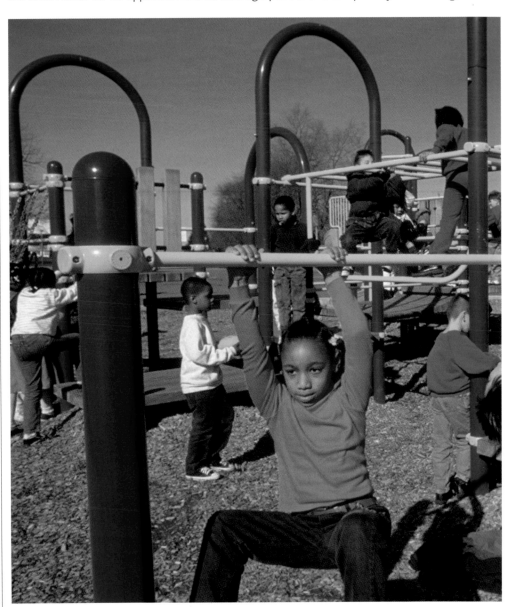

▲ *A stitch is a common feature in the typical rough-and-tumble of childhood playtime. Impetuously returning to play too soon after eating is the most usual cause, but any burst of sudden exercise may be enough to bring on the stabbing pain of a stitch.*

2086

is usually more of a nuisance than a serious complaint. There are, however, some diseases that have symptoms which can be confused with a stitch. For this reason, any persistent pain that resembles a stitch should be reported to a doctor (see Cramp).

## How a stitch develops

A stitch has very localized effects, because it is confined solely to the muscles involved in breathing. These are the intercostal muscles between the ribs, which help the rib cage expand and contract; and the diaphragm, which is a sheet of muscle covering the whole of the base of the rib cage. When a breath is taken in, the muscles of the diaphragm contract, pushing the muscle sheet flat; on breathing out, the muscles relax and the diaphragm assumes a domelike shape.

When a stitch comes on, a cramp occurs in the intercostal muscles or the diaphragm, or both. If the intercostal muscles are involved, the pain is usually toward the front of the chest. The effect of this kind of stitch is to make breathing painful. A stabbing pain is felt when a breath is taken in because the muscles cannot contract properly, and it may also be difficult to catch the breath (see Breathing).

When the diaphragm is involved in a stitch, the pain is usually felt at the side of the body. The cramp causes the diaphragm to develop a type of crease. Again, breathing is painful, with the pain bridging the gap between breaths so that to the sufferer it feels continuous. The pain is felt in the side, rather than at the actual site of the problem, because of the way in which the body's nerves are distributed (see Nervous System).

## Exercise and stitch

In common with other forms of cramp, a stitch usually occurs during or after strenuous exercise. It is caused by an inadequate blood supply to the breathing muscles, due to diversion of blood to other parts of the body; by constriction of the blood vessels supplying that part of the body; or by failure of the blood vessels to stretch and so supply sufficient blood during exercise.

During anaerobic exercise such as weight lifting, when the muscles work in short sharp bursts of intense activity, the muscles do not get sufficient oxygen, and there is a buildup of waste products, such as lactic acid, which causes muscle fatigue and cramps that are similar to a stitch (see Aerobics).

A stitch is most likely to develop if exercise is taken immediately after a meal, or if the body's resources are overstretched. However, with regular exercise, the stitches become fewer as the blood vessels widen and become more elastic to take a greater blood flow.

No matter how fit someone may be, exercising after meals can cause a stitch to develop because there is no way of preventing blood from being diverted to the digestive system. It is prudent to always leave a gap of at least an hour after a meal before taking any strenuous exercise.

### Dealing with a stitch

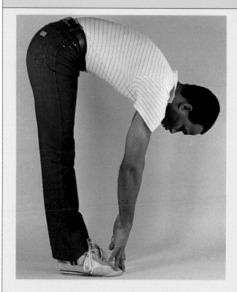

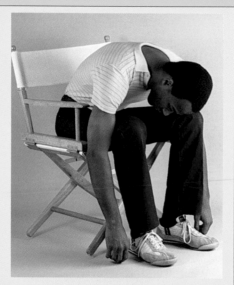

**If you feel a stitch coming on, stop whatever exercise you are doing and bend down and touch your toes. This action effectively eases the cramp out of the muscles.**

**If this fails to work, sit down and bend over so that your head is between your knees. Relax and breathe slowly and deeply. The stitch should then quickly disappear.**

## Full stomach

A weakness in the diaphragm may also lead to a stitch after even the slightest exercise, or just after a heavy meal and without doing any exercise at all. What happens in this case is that a full stomach presses on the diaphragm and causes it to bulge upward. Regurgitation from the stomach up into the esophagus can cause a severe chest pain (see Heartburn).

## Treatment of a stitch

The best way to deal with an ordinary stitch is first to stop exercising, and then to bend down and touch the toes. This action stretches the diaphragm and intercostal muscles and so stops the muscular spasm that is causing the stitch. If this is not effective, it is worth sitting down, relaxing, and trying to breathe in and out as deeply as possible, while keeping the head down between the knees. This action should help to stretch the muscles and stop the spasm that is causing the cramp.

## Causes for confusion

A pain which is similar to a stitch, but which is not related to exercise and is generally more persistent than normal, can be a sign of serious illness and should never be ignored.

Illnesses that result in stitchlike pains include pleurisy, inflammation of the diaphragm caused by infection through bacteria or viruses, and problems of the spleen or colon.

Accordingly, a pain which initially feels like a stitch, but which is particularly associated with severe pains in the chest or abdomen, should be brought to the attention of a doctor without delay.

*See also:* **Blood; Diaphragm; Exercise; Pain; Ribs**

# Stomach

**What happens when people have their stomach removed? Can they eat normally, and what happens to their digestion?**

Usually only part of the stomach is removed. This can still affect them in many ways, however, and they usually find that they feel full after a small meal and have to eat little and often. They must see a doctor regularly as, in the long term, they may become anemic and develop other nutritional deficiencies. If the whole stomach is removed (this is not always necessary), they have more severe symptoms and will require regular injections of vitamin B12, since the stomach secretes a factor necessary for the natural absorption of this vitamin.

**How big is the stomach and does its size vary?**

It can vary considerably in size. It may be the size of a large pear or so large that it almost reaches the pelvis. Eating a lot of food may cause it to enlarge and a blockage to the outlet of the stomach could have the same effect. However, when someone is said to have a large stomach, this usually means that the abdomen is fat.

**Is the stomach ever empty, or does it always contain some food?**

Food entering the stomach takes an hour or so to pass into the intestines. After this, apart from a small amount of digestive juice, the stomach is empty.

**Is drinking alcohol on an empty stomach harmful?**

Alcohol would be more quickly absorbed into the bloodstream, so it is inadvisable to drink alcohol without food, since it can damage the lining of the stomach, causing inflammation and bleeding.

**The stomach is the body's natural reservoir. It holds the food we eat and begins the digestive process. The products of digestion are then absorbed through the intestinal lining into the bloodstream and circulated.**

The stomach is a muscular bag situated in the upper left part of the abdomen. It is connected at its upper end to the esophagus, and at its lower end to the duodenum. The wall of the stomach consists of a thick layer of muscle lined with a special membrane called epithelium. The stomach acts as a reservoir for food. The lining membrane produces a juice that contains acid and enzymes to break down the food and aid digestion. In the stomach the food is mixed with digestive juices until it forms a pulp, called chyme, which is then moves into the duodenum. At the junction between the stomach and the duodenum there is a ring of muscle, the pyloric sphincter or pylorus. The pylorus closes if large pieces of food leave the stomach; then anti-peristaltic waves in the stomach wall churn the food pieces back into the stomach for further enzyme and acid treatment. Chyme is then pushed along the intestines to be further digested and absorbed (see Digestive System).

## Common problems

Vomiting occurs when the stomach contracts forcibly. When this happens, the contents of the stomach may be ejected upward into the esophagus, an action known as vomiting. Vomiting can have several causes: any disturbance of the central nervous system, which controls the contraction of the stomach; an irritation of the lining of the stomach; or an obstruction of the

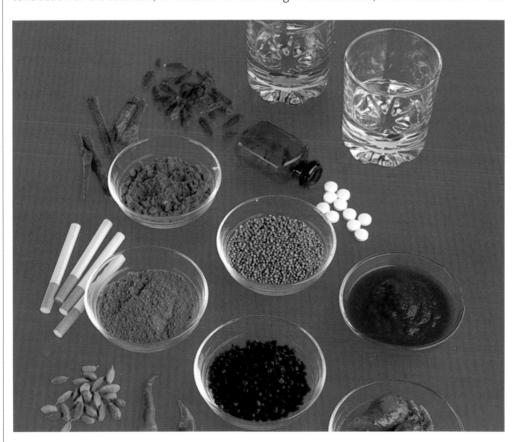

▲ *Stomach problems such as gastritis or ulcers can flare up for a variety of reasons, but perhaps most frequently as a result of eating spicy food, drinking alcohol, and taking certain drugs.*

outflow from the lower end of the stomach (see Vomiting). Often, vomiting is due to a common condition known as gastroenteritis, in which the lining of the stomach becomes inflamed as a result of a viral infection, eating spicy foods, drinking alcohol, taking certain drugs, or stress. A mild attack of gastritis produces symptoms of nausea, vomiting, and occasionally some pain in the upper abdomen. Severe attacks can result in bleeding from the stomach lining.

The treatment of gastritis is to remove the cause and to drink bland fluids. Drugs which prevent vomiting may be prescribed by a doctor. Gastritis, however, is usually a self-limiting condition once the primary cause has been removed.

## Gastric ulcers

Ulcers occur in the stomach when there is a local failure of the mucous layer that protects the lining and prevents it from being affected by the strong acid and enzymes naturally present in the gastric juices (see Ulcers). The spiral germ *Helicobacter pylori* is an important factor in causing chronic gastritis and promoting stomach ulcers. *H. pylori* infection can be detected by a urea breath test, by antibody tests, by stool tests, or by endoscopy biopsy. The acid can erode the mucosal layer, then penetrate the muscle layer. This may lead to perforation of the stomach wall, causing an ulcer. Many gastric ulcers appear to be present for many years before medical advice is sought, because of scarring and fibrous tissue around the ulcer.

People who develop gastric ulcers do not have a high level of acid in the stomach, unlike those people who develop duodenal ulcers. In fact, some patients with gastric ulcers have a low level of acid secretion.

## Symptoms and dangers

Gastric ulcers are most commonly found on the upper aspect of the stomach (the lesser curve). They tend to appear, grow bigger, then disappear. Not all the causes of gastric ulcers are known, but spicy foods, alcohol, smoking, and stress are contributory factors.

The symptoms include burning pain, which comes shortly after eating; nausea; and sometimes weight loss. There may be episodes of these symptoms followed by long periods without any symptoms at all. If a gastric ulcer is left untreated for a long period of time, several things can happen. First, if the ulcer is situated over a main blood

**STOMACH: SITE AND STRUCTURE**

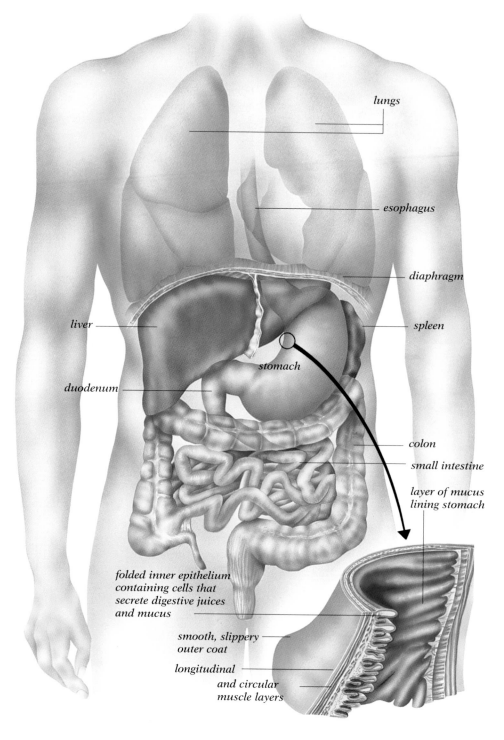

lungs

esophagus

diaphragm

liver

spleen

stomach

duodenum

colon

small intestine

layer of mucus lining stomach

folded inner epithelium containing cells that secrete digestive juices and mucus

smooth, slippery outer coat

longitudinal and circular muscle layers

**Section through stomach wall**

▲ *The stomach is situated higher up in the body than most people think—in fact, it is found just under the diaphragm. It is a muscular bag with a smooth, slippery outer coat and a corrugated inner lining that is protected from its own acidic digestive juices by a layer of mucus.*

## Questions and Answers

**My husband is 60 years old and he has started getting persistent indigestion pains. Antacids, such as milk of magnesia, do not really seem to be helping much. What should he do next?**

It is important for someone of his age who has developed persistent indigestion to have investigations to make sure that he has not developed a stomach tumor. Your doctor should arrange for him to have a number of tests, which will probably include a gastroscopy. The latter enables the doctor to see into the stomach by means of a flexible telescopic instrument (a gastroscope) passed through the mouth and esophagus.

**Is it normal to lose weight with an ulcer?**

It depends on what sort of ulcer it is. If the ulcer is in the duodenum, eating relieves the pain and the patient may put on weight. However, if the ulcer is in the stomach, eating causes pain so the patient tends to lose weight because he or she is afraid to eat.

**I had an attack of vomiting and loss of appetite. My doctor said it was gastric flu. Is this possible?**

Yes. You probably developed a viral infection of the stomach, causing its lining to become inflamed. However, there is no way of proving that this is what it was. The symptoms of viral gastritis, as it should be called, are usually short-lived, and respond to simple measures such as drinking bland liquids, and possibly taking tablets to prevent vomiting.

**Does a stomach tumor always cause pain?**

No. Sometimes there is no pain at all. The patient simply notices a loss of appetite, or loss of weight. In fact, pain can often confuse the issue, and sometimes leads to a misdiagnosis if the patient is simply thought to have attacks of indigestion.

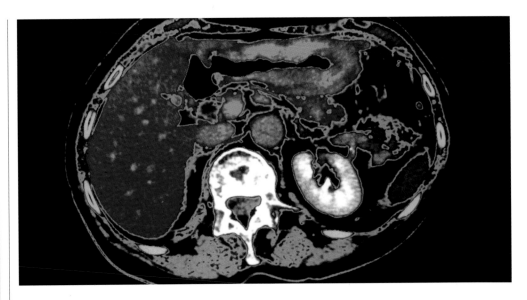

▲ *Computer-assisted imaging (CT) uses X-ray beams to produce a cross-sectional picture of a stomach. The tomogram produced shows that cancer is present.*

vessel supplying the wall of the stomach, it may erode through the blood vessel, leading to a massive hemorrhage (see Hemorrhage). Second, the ulcer can perforate the wall of the stomach; the stomach contents can then leak out into the peritoneal cavity, causing peritonitis. Third, repeated attempts at healing the ulcer may lead to scarring and contraction of the tissues around the ulcer. This may eventually produce a narrowing in the middle of the stomach so that it assumes an hourglass appearance.

### Treatment

Diagnosis of a gastric ulcer is usually made by means of a gastroscopy to ensure that the ulcer is benign. Eradication of *Helicobacter pylori* is the first step; this is done with antibiotics. Recently developed drugs, such as proton pump inhibitors, are so effective in controlling gastric acid production that surgery for gastric ulceration is now required much less often than formerly.

### Cancer of the stomach

Gastric cancer is one of the most common malignant tumors, and it affects more men than women. It can start as a small ulcer or as a small polyp and grows bigger to obstruct the passage of food through the stomach. Because the tumor involves the lining of the stomach, patients may lose blood into the stomach, and anemia may signal that there is a problem.

Other symptoms are constant nausea and loss of appetite, and weight loss. Pain may develop in the upper part of the abdomen. Because the pain can be similar to that caused by a benign gastric or duodenal ulcer, patients are often treated for a long time with antacids with no relief of symptoms.

It is for this reason that any patient over the age of about 50 years with indigestion should be treated with caution. If he or she does not respond quickly to conventional treatment for indigestion, further investigation of the case will be essential (see Indigestion).

Like a benign ulcer, gastric cancer is usually diagnosed by a gastroscopy. Early diagnosis improves the overall outlook of the treatment. Whenever possible the treatment of gastric cancer involves surgical removal of the tumor, which often involves removing the whole stomach. Patients who have had their stomach, or a major portion of it, removed cannot eat large meals, but in other respects may live a normal life. They need yearly checkups, since they are more likely to develop anemia and nutritional disturbances, which can usually be corrected.

Sometimes the outlet of the stomach, the pyloric canal, becomes blocked, leading to a buildup of stomach contents followed by profuse vomiting. In infants this can occur as a result of overgrowth of the muscle in this region. In adults, it is caused either by a cancerous growth or by a long-standing duodenal ulcer, which has caused fibrous scarring.

*See also:* **Cancer; Gastroenteritis**

# Stomach pump

A stomach pump is a device for washing out harmful substances from the stomach before they are absorbed, usually in cases of drug overdose. Although it is a term in common parlance, no actual pumping is involved.

When a stomach pump is used, a tube is passed from the mouth to the stomach and water is passed down it. The water is siphoned out or aspirated, bringing with it the unwanted substance, usually tablets taken in overdose. The procedure has to be done before they can be absorbed and do any harm to the patient. The procedure is known medically as gastric lavage.

## When it is needed

Drug overdose, either accidental or deliberate, is a common cause of hospital admission. Accidental overdoses often occur if children swallow their parents' pills or household remedies, such as aspirin, by mistake (see Overdoses). In adults, it is most likely that the overdose has been taken as a deliberate suicide attempt, although not all people who take overdoses actually intend to die. Whatever the reason, acts of self-poisoning are common. The drugs used are not only those obtained on prescription, but ones which can be bought over the counter, such as aspirin and acetaminophen. Other drugs commonly used for overdoses are tranquilizers and antidepressants (see Tranquilizers). The drugs are often taken in combination, and very often alcohol is also consumed.

## Intensive care

Emergency room treatment aims to keep alive a patient who has taken an overdose. This means that it is more important for the trauma team to check and maintain vital life functions, rather than immediately try to wash out the drug from the stomach (see Emergencies). They must clear and maintain an airway, perhaps by inserting a tube to assist breathing, or even by putting the patient on a machine called a respirator which will help him or her to breathe. It is also important for doctors to check blood pressure, and give drugs if this has fallen dangerously low. These in

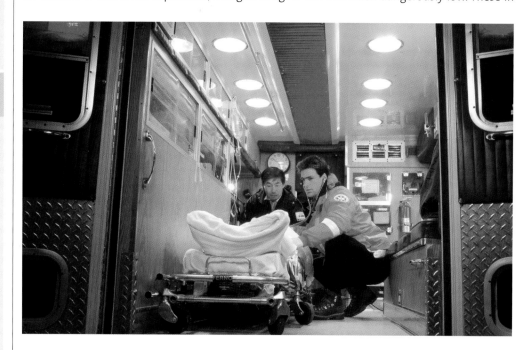

▲ *In dealing with an emergency case of drug overdose, the first priority is to ensure the patient's vital life functions. Drugs may be given to help stabilize the blood pressure, and blankets will prevent hypothermia.*

## Questions and Answers

**Who actually performs a stomach washout procedure?**

A stomach pump is used at the direction of a doctor and usually inserted by a nurse who is experienced in the technique.

**When is a stomach pump commonly used?**

It is most often used in the treatment of people who have taken overdoses of such drugs as tranquilizers or antidepressants. It is particularly useful as a treatment up to four hours after the drug has been taken, but it is often used up to 10 or even 12 hours afterward.

**Is there a danger of internal damage from a stomach pump?**

This is unlikely. A similar principle is involved when a patient has abdominal surgery. The same kind of tube of a smaller size is inserted into the stomach so that secretions can be sucked out while the intestines are not functioning. Likewise, a patient who is unconscious will be fed by a tube inserted through the nose and passed into the stomach. It causes no harm to the patient but enables him or her to receive a normal diet in liquid form.

**Will the normal digestive process be upset after the stomach has been washed out?**

Usually a patient who has taken an overdose does not feel like eating, and the patient may not be able to eat if he or she is unconscious. By the time consciousness is regained, the digestive processes should be restored, without any damage.

**Why is lukewarm water always used for a washout?**

Quite simply, the water must be the same temperature as the body. If too hot, it could burn the internal organs; if too cold it may cause shock.

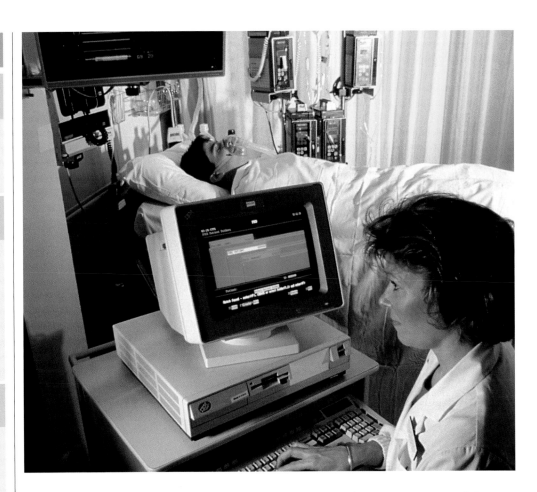

▲ *Washing out a drug from the stomach may not be an adequate treatment. If the poison has had sufficient time to pass into the bloodstream, prolonged treatment in an intensive care unit may still be required.*

turn can cause irregularity in the heart's action, and this must also be checked and corrected. The patient may become very cold (develop hypothermia); this must be treated promptly.

The drug that has been taken must be identified. For this reason, it is extremely important that anyone who accompanies the patient to the hospital takes along the empty pill container. In cases of doubt, physicians should take samples of blood and urine for drug analysis (see Specimens). When these procedures have been carried out, doctors will decide whether or not the use of a stomach pump is appropriate.

### Use of the stomach pump

A stomach pump should be used fairly soon after the overdose has been taken: that is, before the drug has disappeared from the stomach and been absorbed into the intestines. This usually implies that a washout is most likely to be effective within four hours after the drug has been taken. The decision whether or not to use a stomach pump is based on evidence of the type and number of pills taken. If someone has swallowed only two or three pills as a symbolic gesture there is little point in subjecting him or her to a stomach pump. It may be worth attempting to remove certain drugs, such as acetaminophen, up to 12 hours after they have been taken.

### Dangers and precautions

The chief danger of the stomach pump procedure is that fluid may accidentally be aspirated into the lungs and may cause pneumonia (see Pneumonia). It should never be used on any patient who has taken paraffin, or strong acid, or alkali solutions (these can do more damage as they are siphoned out). It is also dangerous to perform the procedure on an unconscious person without establishing an airway into his or her windpipe. Afterward, some people may suffer from chest complications (see Chest). It may be possible to induce a conscious patient to vomit by means of a special drug called an emetic, and avoid the need for a stomach pump (see Emetics; Vomiting).

## HOW THE STOMACH PUMP IS USED

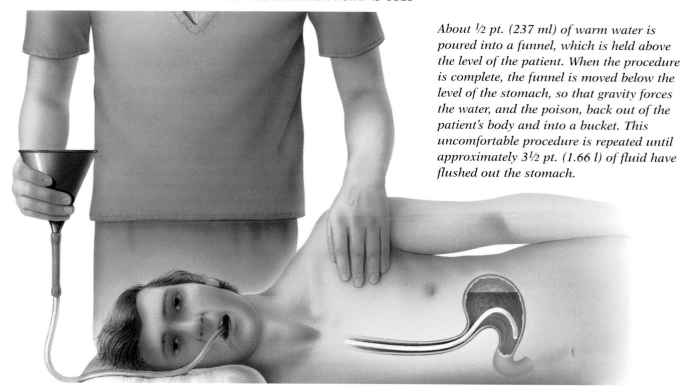

About ½ pt. (237 ml) of warm water is poured into a funnel, which is held above the level of the patient. When the procedure is complete, the funnel is moved below the level of the stomach, so that gravity forces the water, and the poison, back out of the patient's body and into a bucket. This uncomfortable procedure is repeated until approximately 3½ pt. (1.66 l) of fluid have flushed out the stomach.

Emetics are considered by some to be very useful in treating children who have taken overdoses, but should never be used with any patient who is drowsy, drugged, or unconscious.

If doctors do decide to use a stomach pump on an unconscious patient, it is essential that the windpipe or trachea is blocked off so that no stomach contents can enter the lungs. This is done by means of an endotracheal tube (a tube placed in the trachea and then sealed off with an air-filled balloon).

### Effectiveness

The reliability of the stomach pump technique has been debated by doctors for many years, but essentially it depends on the experience of the people who decide on and perform the procedure.

In addition, it should be pointed out that, since the use of the barbiturate family of sedatives has declined, the number of patients who actually die from overdose has fallen considerably. In one survey of 236 patients admitted to a major hospital, not one died after admission. This group of people had often taken tranquilizers, antidepressants, acetaminophen, and aspirin, sometimes in combinations of two or more. Less than 3 percent had taken barbiturates. In the majority of cases a stomach pump was used, and it was, as a conclusion, recommended for the treatment of patients who have taken more than 10 tablets, particularly those of the aspirin family.

One of the great advantages of putting a tube into the stomach is that not only can the stomach then be washed out but substances can also be introduced that are able to slow down the absorption of poisonous drugs. For example, a special form of activated charcoal will inhibit the absorption of acetaminophen, and a special chemical binding agent called desferrioxamine is used in the case of iron tablets, which are sometimes taken accidentally by young children. The decision to use the stomach pump should really be based on the

### Stomach pump procedure

The patient is positioned with his or her head down, and a rubber tube, about ⅜ in. (1 cm) in diameter and 18 in. (45 cm) long, is passed into the stomach via the mouth.

A funnel is attached to the end of the tube; its position is checked and ½ pt. (250 ml) of lukewarm water introduced.

This is left for two or three minutes, then allowed to flow out by a siphon action.

The process is repeated until up to 3½ pt. (2 liters) of water have been used. The fluid is run out by gravity.

doctor's interpretation as to whether or not the patient has taken potentially lethal quantities of a drug. A frequent problem is that the patient, if conscious, may not give a clear account of the type and quantity of drug he or she has taken. For example, the patient may say that he or she has taken only a mild tranquilizer, in which case it would be safe not to use the stomach pump. The doctor may, however, have reason to doubt the patient's accuracy, and, in such cases, it is clearly in the patient's interest for the procedure to be carried out, unpleasant though it may be.

The stomach pump therefore plays an essential role in emergency medical management of a patient who has taken a drug overdose, although the most important factor in saving his or her life is immediate access to intensive life support .

*See also:* **Hypothermia; Suicide**

# Strangulation

**Questions and Answers**

**Internal strangulation occurs when the constriction of a tubular structure of the body, such as the windpipe, intestine, or a blood vessel, prevents normal functioning and circulation. In some forms, it is potentially fatal.**

The word "strangulation" conjures up an image of someone struggling desperately for breath while another person grips him or her tightly about the throat. There is, however, another meaning, since strangulation or compression of other parts of the body can also take place. Areas of the intestine or sections of blood vessels in the limbs, for example, can be strangulated so that circulation is interrupted and function is impaired, and an inadequate amount of blood reaches the area (a condition called ischemia), possibly leading to death of the affected tissue (see Gangrene). The outcome is extremely serious, and urgent surgery must be performed.

### Intestinal strangulation

Intestinal strangulation occurs when the blood flow to the intestine is interrupted, leading to swelling (edema), discoloration (cyanosis), and gangrene. This condition is usually caused by a hernia (see Hernia); the telescoping of a short segment of bowel into itself (called intussusception); or a twisting of the intestine onto itself to cause an intestinal obstruction (called volvulus). Intussusception occurs mainly in babies and small children, and is characterized by abdominal pain, vomiting, and bloody mucus in the stool. A barium enema (see Enema) can be used to confirm the diagnosis, and the obstruction is corrected surgically.

If a case of volvulus is left untreated, the section of obstructed intestine involved will die; peritonitis, which is inflammation of the peritoneum— the covering of the abdominal wall—will occur; the intestine will rupture; and the patient may die. Early signs of intestinal strangulation resemble those of intestinal obstruction: severe pain, vomiting of fecal matter, dehydration, failure of the contents of the intestine to pass through the bowel, and abdominal distension. Peritonitis, shock, and the presence of a tender mass in the abdomen are also found with

**Can a hernia be strangulated?**

Yes. It is a dangerous condition and must be dealt with urgently. What happens is that a loop of intestine passes through a narrow opening in the abdominal wall and its blood supply is at risk. Because veins are more easily compressed than arteries, blood can get into the loop but can't get out. Unless the loop is quickly restored to its original position, with its blood supply, tension will increase until the arterial supply is cut off. Soon after, the tissues of the loop will die.

**What happens if a strangulated hernia becomes gangrenous?**

When any part of the body is deprived of blood, it soon dies (becomes gangrenous). The only possible treatment is to cut away all of the dead gangrenous tissue and join together the healthy cut ends of the intestine.

**My baby was born with a bowel obstruction and had surgery. Why?**

Doctors call this unusual condition volvulus neonatorum. During fetal development, part of the intestine twists around itself because it is not held together tightly enough, causing an intestinal obstruction. Immediate surgical correction is needed to prevent the affected portion of the intestine from becoming gangrenous.

**Can a baby be strangled by its own umbilical cord during birth?**

No. The cord may get twisted around the baby's neck, and this can cause fetal distress and even death. It is not strangulation that is the problem, but cord compression, which occurs when a loop of the cord comes out before the baby is born. Cord accidents indicate urgent cesarean section.

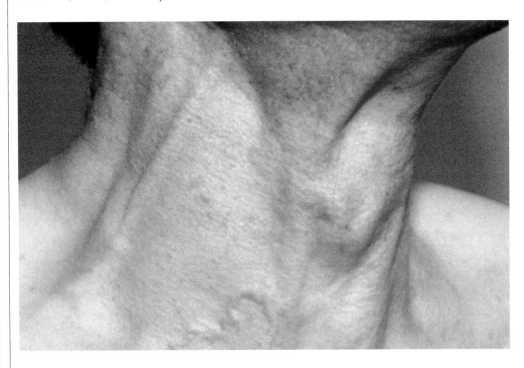

▲ *External strangulation occurs when violent pressure is exerted on the neck's carotid artery, starving the brain of oxygen. Similarly, internal strangulations occur when the body's organs become deprived of blood, usually as a result of hernias.*

intestinal strangulation. The position of the intestinal obstruction and its cause can be revealed by X-ray examination. Treatment includes the removal of intestinal contents using a special tube and sometimes surgical repair. In the case of intestinal strangulation, surgery is always required.

## Hernias

A hernia, or rupture, occurs when an organ or part of an organ becomes displaced through the lining of the cavity in which it is normally situated. One of the most common types of hernia occurs when a section of intestine protrudes through the front wall of the abdominal cavity, often as a result of muscular strain or injury.

The most feared complication of hernia is strangulation. Like all other organs of the body, the intestine has a blood supply; arteries carry blood to the intestine and veins carry blood away. Arteries are high-pressure vessels whereas veins are low-pressure vessels. Because of this, the walls of the veins are much thinner and softer than those of the arteries. When a loop of intestine passes through a constricted opening, as in a hernia, the blood continues to pass into the loop through the arteries. However, constriction on the easily compressed veins soon means that the amount of blood in the loop increases. This causes the hernia to swell, and the swelling in turn causes further constriction and increased compression of the veins.

Eventually, the return of blood through the veins stops, there is massive swelling, and soon the arterial blood supply is also cut off. The result is a strangulated hernia, which is a highly dangerous condition. Any part of the body deprived of blood soon dies and becomes gangrenous. In the case of a strangulated hernia, the passage of the normal intestinal contents is also totally obstructed.

## Surgical treatment

Surgery is the only treatment possible in the case of gangrene following a strangulated hernia. The situation cannot be remedied simply by replacing the loop into the abdomen, which could be fatal. The gangrenous piece of intestine must be removed surgically, and the two healthy cut ends joined. Sometimes, the two cut ends cannot be joined up immediately and the upper cut end must be brought outside of the body through an artificial opening in the abdominal wall. This is called a colostomy (see Colostomy), or a jejunostomy, depending on which part of the intestine is involved.

## Hemorrhoids

Strangulation can also affect parts of the body other than the intestines. Veins that become swollen and twisted in the region of the anus and lower rectum are called hemorrhoids (piles), and are often painful and bleeding (see Hemorrhoids; Rectum). When hemorrhoids pass outside the anal opening they are described as prolapsed. They can become trapped by the anal sphincter, the tight

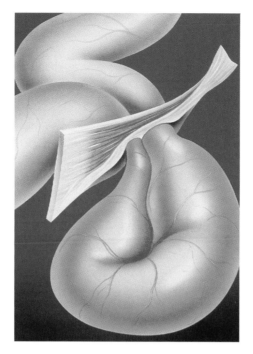

▲ *In this illustration of an intestinal hernia, the intestine (orange) has burst through the abdominal wall. The protruding region (pink) has impaired blood supply and requires urgent surgical treatment if gangrene (tissue death) is to be prevented.*

muscular band that closes the anal opening, and their blood supply can be cut off. Anal piles are sometimes deliberately strangulated: tight rubber bands are used to encircle the hemorrhoids and cut off their blood supply so that they fall away in time.

## Intussusception

Intussusception is a condition in which a segment of the intestine slides inside the adjoining segment in the manner of a naval telescope being closed. This process is called invagination, and it usually occurs at a point in the intestine where the lower part of the small intestine (the ileum) joins the wider large intestine (the colon). Understandably, invagination can occur more easily at this junction than at any other point in the entire intestine. Intussusception is the most common cause of strangulation and blockage of the intestine in the first two years of life. Surprisingly, it is three times as common in male babies as in females.

In most cases, the condition occurs for no discernible reason. It can start as a result of constipation, with hard fecal material in the intestine (see Constipation). Occasionally, swelling lymphoid patches in the lining of the small intestine are pushed by moving bowel contents into the colon. Small benign fatty tumors of the intestine called lipomas can act in the same way. Intussusception is a fairly common feature of cystic fibrosis (see Cystic Fibrosis). To understand how intussusception causes strangulation of the intestine, it is necessary to appreciate that the coils of the intestine are suspended from the inner back wall of the abdomen by a thin membrane called the mesentery. The mesentery contains the arteries and veins that carry blood to and from the intestine. When the intestine telescopes, part of the mesentery, with its blood vessels, is dragged into the wider part of the large intestine

The first result is that the veins, in which the pressure of blood is lower than in the arteries, become compressed. Therefore, blood being pumped into the walls of the intestine through the arteries is unable to get out, so the affected part of the intestine quickly swells up with the increased volume of fluid. The resulting increase in compression closes off the arteries also.

Any part of the body that is wholly deprived of its blood supply must necessarily die. This is a critical state of affairs because dead bowel will soon perforate, releasing the highly contaminated contents into the sterile area in the peritoneal sac that surrounds the intestine. The result is infection of the peritoneal membrane, a condition known as peritonitis. Unless urgently treated by surgery, peritonitis is usually fatal.

Intussusception is thus a surgical emergency that will tolerate no delay. Obviously, it is extremely important to avoid intestinal perforation and peritonitis if at all possible, so the earlier the diagnosis is made the better. The symptoms are characteristic. The baby suddenly develops attacks of screaming and drawing up of the knees. Soon after this vomiting nearly always begins. Within 12 hours

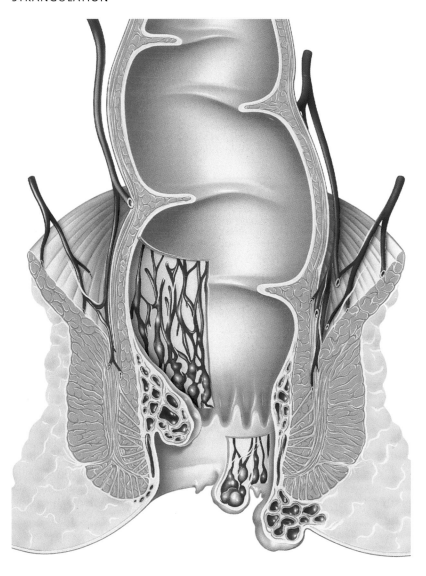

▲ *Illustration of a section through a human anus showing internal and external hemorrhoids (lower center, blue)—swollen and strangulated veins.*

## Other types of strangulation

An unusual cause of strangulation is the growth of tumors inside the neck (see Neck). Cancers of the thyroid gland (see Thyroid), for example, can grow extremely rapidly and can spread locally to compress adjacent structures. This can lead to strangulation by compression of the great blood vessels of the neck, or even by compression of the windpipe or voice box. Pressure on the two main arteries of the neck, the carotids, deprives the brain of blood and leads to loss of consciousness. Pressure on the great veins prevents the return of blood from the brain and has the same effect. The term "carotid" and the word "garrote" come from the Greek word meaning "to stupefy," and it is clear that the Greeks were aware that strangulation had its effect at least partly by compression of these arteries.

When neck tumors press on and obstruct the airway, an emergency tracheotomy (a surgical operation to allow breathing that makes a new opening called a tracheostomy in the windpipe) may be necessary (see Tracheostomy). Urgent surgery to remove the tumor will also be necessary.

Strangulation of the heart (see Heart Disease) is a very rare condition that can occur when an opening in the fibrous bag that surrounds the heart (the pericardial sac) allows part of the heart to herniate through.

As a result of severe abdominal injuries—in automobile accidents, for example—various abdominal organs can herniate through the diaphragm and into the chest, where they may strangulate.

Similarly, if there are severe head injuries (see Head and Head Injuries) that involve bleeding in the skull, the increased pressure can force the brain to herniate downward through the large opening at the base of the skull (the foramen magnum), compressing part of the brain called the brain stem, and causing fatal strangulation. This complication is one of the most serious intermediate and late effects of head injury and may occur with or without fracture of the skull.

Typically an injured person is briefly unconscious and then recovers, but later within hours or days develops a severe headache with vomiting, drowsiness, and confusion, and then lapses again into unconsciousness (see Unconsciousness). This dangerous situation, which is inevitably fatal unless treated, is the result of the formation of a blood clot (hematoma) on the outer surface of the brain that increases in size. Because the skull is unyielding, the brain is gradually forced downward. The vital centers for respiration and heartbeat are in the brain stem, and compression of these, or of their supplying blood vessels, against the edge of the foramen magnum is a common cause of death.

This form of strangulation of nerve tissue and small blood vessels is remediable only by neurosurgery. The procedure involves folding back a flap of scalp, temporarily removing a rectangular area of the vault of the skull to expose the hematoma, sucking it out, securing and closing any bleeding points, and replacing the bone and scalp. Performed in time, such surgery is lifesaving.

**See also: Anus; Surgery**

or so the baby passes blood and mucus in its stools. The infant's abdomen is distended and is extremely tender to touch. Careful examination of the abdomen will reveal a sausage-shaped mass; the thickened and swollen length of double bowel.

Attempts are usually made to relieve intussusception by nonsurgical means. This is done by giving a barium enema drip, through the rectum, without applying more pressure than is provided by keeping the barium container at a height of approximately 3 feet (1 m). Applied in time, the gentle, internal hydrostatic pressure of the barium solution will reverse the intussusception in 75 percent of cases. Barium is opaque to X ray, so success can be proved by observing on X ray the free flow of barium back into the small intestine (see X rays).

If this method fails, there is no choice but open surgery to pull out the segment of telescoped intestine, and, if necessary, to remove a length of necrotic (dead) bowel and join the free ends together. Unrelieved intussusception is almost always fatal.

# Streptococcus

**How did the streptococcus bacterium get its name?**

A coccus is a roughly spherical germ named after the Greek word *kokkos,* meaning "a berry." Germs reproduce by growing longer and then splitting into two. When streptococci do this, the daughter cells tend to stick together to form a chain like a string of beads. When this appearance was first noted under the microscope by the German surgeon Albert Billroth, he decided to call them after the Greek word for "a chain." However, he was mistaken as to the meaning of the word, since *strepto* means "twisted," but no one objected, so the name stuck.

**Is it true that there are a lot of streptococci in people's mouths?**

Yes, billions, but most of these are species that do not cause serious disease and many of them are entirely harmless. *Streptococcus mutans* in tooth plaque, however, is one of the principal causes of tooth decay, and *Streptococcus viridans* can cause serious infections of the heart lining and valves (bacterial endocarditis) in people who have had rheumatic fever if these germs get into the bloodstream during dental treatment.

**What exactly is a strep throat and why is it more serious than a regular sore throat?**

Most of the germs that cause sore throat are of reasonably low virulence, but *Streptococcus pyogenes,* which is the principal disease-causing streptococcus, can cause a dangerous infection. The danger is not so much to the throat itself as to the body generally in the aftermath of the infection. Strep throat may lead to a potentially serious kidney disorder called glomerulonephritis and to a joint and heart disorder called rheumatic fever.

Of the many different streptococcal species, only a few cause disease in humans. Those that do can be very dangerous, causing serious illness or even death, but most, if diagnosed early, can be effectively treated with antibiotics.

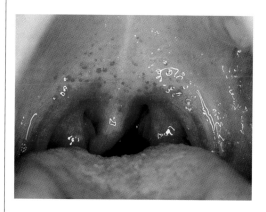

▲ *The streptococcus bacterium causes small red spots to form on the soft palate at the back of the mouth in the condition known as strep throat.*

A streptococcus is a spherical or ovoid bacterium about a thousandth of a millimeter in diameter. Under a microscope, individual streptococci look the same as staphylococci (see Staphylococcus), but when they have been reproducing, streptococci remain in pairs or form characteristic short or long chains. Unlike many bacteria, they are incapable of independent movement and do not form spores. Streptococci stain deep blue with standard Gram's stain; they are said to be "gram-positive." Streptococci are found normally in the mouth and intestines of humans. They also occur in dairy products and other foods, and in fermenting plant juices. There are at least 85 different species of streptococci but only a few cause disease.

## Streptococcal species

*Streptococcus pyogenes* is a pus-forming bacterium (see Pus) and the most dangerous of all the streptococcal species. It causes impetigo, acute tonsillitis, scarlet fever, the spreading skin infection erysipelas, septic abortion, puerperal fever, necrotizing fasciitis, muscle infection (myositis; see Muscles), and urinary infections. It produces many powerful toxins, some of the most important being hemolysins, which attack and destroy red blood cells. For this reason *S. pyogenes* is also known as a hemolytic streptococcus, or a group A streptococcus.

*Streptococcus mutans* acts on sugar in the mouth to convert it to lactic acid, which, in turn, demineralizes the enamel of the teeth. The bacterium also secretes a high-molecular-weight complex sugar (polysaccharide) that binds streptococci with other materials to form plaque.

*Streptococcus fecalis* is present in large numbers in the lower bowel and contaminates the skin around the anus. It is a common cause of urinary infections, especially in women, whose short urethra allows the streptococci to reach the bladder more easily than in men (see Urethra).

*Streptococcus pneumoniae,* also known as the pneumococcus, is the most common cause, worldwide, of lung inflammation (pneumonia) and infection of the brain coverings (meningitis). This species of streptococcus, however, has a polysaccharide capsule that allows an effective vaccine to be made against it (see Meningitis; Pneumonia).

## Secondary effects of streptococci

The infections caused by *S. pyogenes* are often serious, but will almost always respond to antibiotic treatment (see Antibiotics). However, infection is not the only damage streptococci can cause: when they enter the body the immune system mounts a defense by producing antibodies against them. These are effective in immobilizing and destroying the invading streptococci, but they also have a dangerous secondary effect. Certain tissues in the large joints, in the heart lining, and in the kidneys have features in common with streptococci, so the antibodies, as well as attacking the bacteria, may attack these tissues. This is how rheumatic fever and glomerulonephritis are caused. These are not infections by streptococci, but autoimmune reactions caused by the antibodies provoked by the streptococcal infection.

> *See also:* Bacteria; Impetigo; Rheumatic fever; Sore throat; Throat; Tonsils

# Stress

## Questions and Answers

**Does everyone suffer from feelings of stress?**

Yes. Stress is an integral part of life. However, you have to be clear about what you mean by stress; it is not always unpleasant. For example, participating in, or even watching, competitive games involves considerable stress.

**Is there good stress and bad stress?**

Yes, in a way, but what you call bad stress might be very important to you. It might, for example, result in a lifesaving level of arousal and physical capability. In acute emergencies, people can perform amazing feats of strength or agility that would be impossible without stress.

**Can stress be pleasurable?**

A young stockbroker, tennis player, or champion skier would no doubt say "yes." Many occupations and activities involve pleasurable stress. Stress can be necessary to achieve a certain standard of performance.

**But if stress is damaging, how come all these people don't die from heart attacks?**

Stress can be damaging to some people, but others can withstand enormous strain without suffering any harm. The idea that a lot of stress will inevitably cause heart attacks, ulcers, skin disease, or cancer isn't borne out by the facts.

**So is there no scientific evidence that stress is harmful?**

Yes, severe, acute stress, such as life-threatening situations, can be harmful. Post-traumatic stress disorder is a real medical entity. However, the occasional stresses of minor emergencies are things we can't do without. We need them.

---

**The popular view is that many diseases are caused by stress and, although this view is not universally accepted by doctors, the medical profession is now beginning to acknowledge that some stress can result in sickness.**

The popular medical media have had a wonderful time with stress. For years, writers of books and articles for lay consumption have been stating or implying that almost any organic disorder can be attributed to stress. Such claims have met with a ready public response. Nearly all people are familiar with the unpleasant feeling of being stressed, and it is not surprising that they therefore fear that it may be doing them harm.

One of the reasons for the appeal of the early writing on the subject in the 1960s and 1970s was that it seemed to be new. The term "stress" was unfamiliar. In those days, people were accustomed to talking about strain, and suddenly everyone started to talk about stress instead. These terms come from the field of engineering; they are not widely understood and they are often confused. Stress is the force exerted on a body that tends to cause it to deform. Strain is a measure of the extent to which a body actually is deformed when it is subjected to stress. The terms can, of course, be applied to human bodies in exactly this mechanical way, but when people talk about biological stress they are usually speaking metaphorically, if not always logically.

## The theory of biological stress

The man who brought stress into the limelight was the Austrian-born Canadian physician Hans Selye (1907–1982), whose initial papers on what he called the stress-adaptation syndrome were produced in the early 1950s. Selye was a well-qualified man who studied medicine in Prague, Paris, and Rome before working at McGill University in Montreal, Canada. In 1945 he became director of the Institute for Experimental Medicine and Surgery at the University of Montreal, an institute which he had founded. From then on Selye produced book after book: *The Story of the Adaptation Syndrome* (1952); *The Stress of Life* (1956); *From Dream to Discovery* (1965); *The Case for Supramolecular Biology* (1967); *Stress without Distress* (1974). These books were directed at the general public, and they made Selye and his ideas famous.

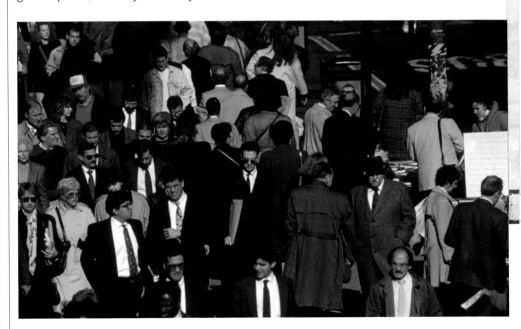

▲ *The hectic yet often monotonous life many people are forced to lead makes a certain amount of stress unavoidable. What can be done, however, is take positive steps, whenever possible, to ensure that these pressures of life are kept to a minimum.*

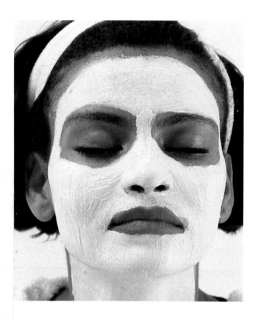

▲ *Physical exercise and pampering of the body, such as indulging in beauty treatments or massage, can help to alleviate the stresses of everyday life.*

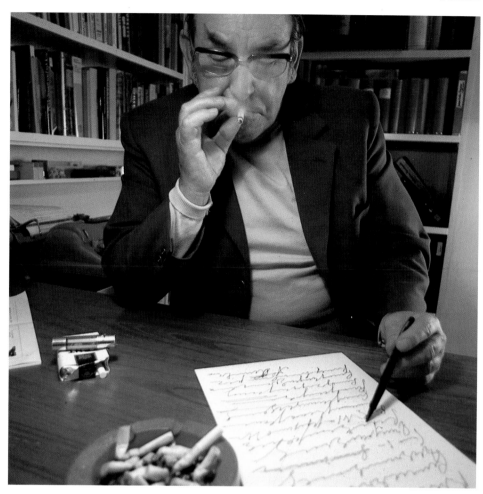

▲ *Different people have different ways of alleviating stress. Some methods, such as excessive smoking or alcohol consumption, are very destructive to the health. Exercise, whether it be jogging, yoga, or even dancing, is a healthier way to combat stress.*

Selye was a physiologist who knew all about the hormonal changes that occur in the body under conditions of anxiety. The production of epinephrine and the steroid hormone cortisol was known to be necessary for survival in fight-or-flight situations (see Hormones). Without these aids to alertness and sudden physical exertion, few primitive humans would have survived to take part in the evolutionary process. So, by natural selection, they became part of people's physical and physiological makeup. None of this was controversial.

Selye first thought of the idea of biological stress when he was a medical student. It occurred to him that all sick patients, however diverse their conditions and symptoms, had this in common: they looked and felt sick. His professor dismissed this idea as childish nonsense. Ten years later, while working at McGill, Selye discovered that rats who were given various damaging injections, or who were kept cold or persistently overworked, developed enlargement of their adrenal glands, the glands that produce epinephrine and cortisol, and often developed stomach ulcers. These rats were showing a general, and identical, reaction to various stress-producing events (stressors). Was this, he wondered, the thing that all sick people had in common?

His further research and thought led him to propose what he called the general adaptation syndrome. Stressors, whatever their nature—physical threat, actual injury, bacterial infection, social or marital problems, perceived danger of any kind—all caused, Selye claimed, much the same effects. The adaptation syndrome was divided into three parts: the alarm stage (previously described as the fight-or-flight reaction); the resistance, or adaptation, stage; and the exhaustion stage.

The alarm stage features secretion of epinephrine, a rise in the pulse rate (see Pulse) and in blood pressure, rapid breathing, tense muscles, trembling, a feeling of butterflies in the stomach, slowed digestive processes, reduced blood supply to the skin, release of sugar fuel into the blood (see Sugars), and an increase in the clotting power of the blood.

Stressors, Selye suggested, may force the alarm stage to persist for long periods, even for months. If the stressor persists, the level of arousal drops a little but remains high, and in the resistance stage the body tries to repair damage caused in the alarm stage. Eventually, if the stressor persists, the person enters the stage of exhaustion in which he or she becomes highly vulnerable to bodily damage.

Selye was convinced that this mechanism was an important element in the production of such disorders as hardening of the arteries, heart disease, high blood pressure, strokes, stomach and duodenal ulcers, colitis, premenstrual syndrome, diabetes, and arthritis (see Arteries and Artery Disease; Arthritis; Heart Disease; Premenstrual Syndrome; Stroke). Selye called these disorders diseases of adaptation.

## Stressors

Many of these stressors are obvious, and many people feel that they can rate them by the strength of the physiological effects they produce, often by the amount of muscle tension felt in the upper part of the abdomen. These stressors include anxiety, frustration, discomfort, conflict, alarm, excessive ambition—all the things people have come to think of as the stresses of modern life. They also

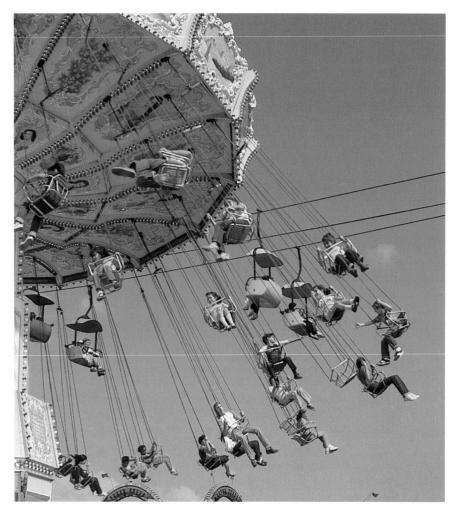

*▲ It is important for people to relax and to get away from their stresses. A trip to the amusement park may be one way of doing this—this activity may look hair-raising, but it will take a person's mind off his or her problems, and this level of fear is considered to be a healthy, invigorating form of stress.*

*▼ Some people let the demands of their job spill into their work breaks. This should be avoided whenever possible, because time to unwind can be vital.*

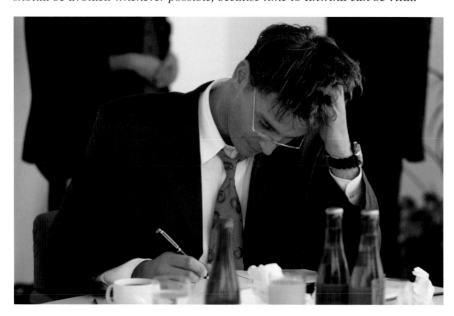

include physical insult to the body, whether from infection, mechanical trauma, burns, radiation, intake of toxic substances, side effects of drugs, exposure to allergens (substances provoking allergic reactions), overcrowding, atmospheric pollution, and so on. There is a real distinction between acute (short and sharp) stress, such as a severe physical assault or a major psychological trauma, and chronic (long-term and less intense) stress, such as being disabled.

One of the most potently perceived stressors is frustration. People's motivation, or goal seeking, is central to their success and satisfaction, and when this is thwarted they are apt to suffer a strong emotional reaction that is felt as frustration. Motivation encompasses the whole spectrum of people's desires, and no one is free from frustration. Thwarting of major motivation may be an almost lifelong process, but people are also beset by numerous small frustrations related to different minor matters. Many people set their goals higher than is appropriate to their innate abilities. In such cases, frustration is likely to be prolonged and may be very severe, causing stress.

In 1967, inspired partly by Selye's work, the psychologists Thomas Holmes and Richard Rahe, working at the University of Washington, came up with a new set of stressors relating to life changes. Selye had already decided that stress was caused by both bad events (distress) and good events (eustress) and that both kinds could cause disease. He postulated that bad stress was usually the more serious because it was nearly always more severe and more persistent than eustress. Holmes and Rahe now came up with a table of events graded in terms of their severity in causing harm. They arbitrarily allotted the figure of 100 to what they considered the most stressful life event—the death of a spouse—and smaller numbers for less severe stressors, such as moving house, going on vacation, or financial troubles.

It is easy to criticize this scheme on the grounds that, for different people, different events can have widely varied significance and, consequently, different stress values. Moreover, most of these events can be quantified over a considerably wide range. Trouble with the boss, for example, might range from a minor disagreement to a major, livelihood-threatening row. Some of the categories actually involve clusters of other changes. Even so, tables of this kind have won a fair measure of acceptance as a guide to the totality of stress suffered by a person.

## Conclusions

What is significant about all this research is that Holmes and Rahe claimed to have found that about 80 percent of people whose total stress events added up to more than 300 points in one year developed serious illness. This compared with about 30 percent of those whose totals were less then 150 in a year.

It has to be said, however, that the ability to withstand stress varies enormously with the person. Some people thrive on stress; other people break down under a minor level. The reasons for this variation remain obscure but may have something to do with personality types (see Personality).

### A-type and B-type personalities

In 1974, the heart specialists Meyer Friedman and Ray H. Rosenman, while studying the causes of heart disease, suggested that many people create their own stress. These are the A-type people: impatient, competitive, driven, and constantly under pressure. A-type people do everything in a hurry. They are always early for appointments, go crazy in traffic jams, and demand perfection of themselves in everything they undertake. The cardiologists concluded that A-type behavior was a more accurate predictor of heart attacks than almost any other combination of factors. B-type people are laid-back, relaxed, patient, easygoing, and are much less prone to heart attacks.

This concept aroused much interest and, for a time, it featured strongly in the medical literature. There were, however, some strong medical criticisms of it, and the initial enthusiasm for the idea was not sustained. Most doctors, however, would admit that there are certainly A-type people around, and that they are more susceptible to certain diseases, especially heart attacks.

### Public and scientific response

Selye's ideas, and those of his followers, have aroused enormous public interest. The response of the medical profession, however, has been muted. Some doctors have accepted the ideas without question. Many who are cautious about adopting new ideas without strong scientific evidence have been more critical. Some voiced strong skepticism; many ignored it in their books and papers or explicitly stated that it was all nonsense.

Selye's assertions have never gained the unequivocal support of the scientific establishment. Even today, when stress has become a household word, his name is conspicuously absent from biographical dictionaries of scientists. There are some reasons for this that are not necessarily related to the intrinsic merit of his ideas. His habit of passing his ideas direct to the public by way of books that ordinary people could understand, for example, did not always endear him to the medical profession, and this may have been the origin of some of the prejudice against him. Doctors like to

| Scale of life event units | |
| --- | --- |
| Death of a spouse | 100 |
| Divorce | 73 |
| Marital separation | 65 |
| Jail term | 63 |
| Marriage | 50 |
| Being fired | 47 |
| Retirement | 45 |
| Pregnancy | 40 |
| New baby | 39 |
| Death of a close friend | 37 |
| Large mortgage | 31 |
| Son or daughter leaving home | 29 |
| In-law trouble | 29 |
| Trouble with employer | 23 |
| Change of residence | 20 |
| Change of school | 20 |
| Vacation | 13 |
| Minor law violation | 11 |

announce medical advances by way of the medical press, where they are subjected to the criticism of their colleagues. This is called peer review. They are not happy when this process is bypassed by those who appeal directly to the public. Selye died without ever having gained full medical acceptance of his ideas.

### What is stress?

The real basis for medical doubts, however, arose from the nature of the subject. For a start, there is the question of definition. What, in short, is stress? It is, of course, entirely subjective. Stress is what people feel, and one person's stress is another person's challenge. What is painfully stressful to one person may be excitingly gratifying to another. Stressors are not, in themselves, stressful. It is the interaction of the stressor and the individual that creates the stress, and people are different in their responses. These points have not always been adequately appreciated, and there has been considerable confusion between cause and effect. Selye himself admitted that his English was not quite good enough for him to appreciate the difference between stress and strain and that he got his terms the wrong way around.

Critics of Holmes's and Rahe's life-event stress factors have pointed out that the results of the research might equally be explained on the hypothesis that people predisposed to physical or psychological disease (see Psychosomatic problems) may be just the kind of people whose lives involve a greater number of stressful changes. Spouses and long-term partners share influences that commonly lead to the development of similar disorders. Also, people with a predisposition to certain types of illness have a higher than average history of being fired from work.

As to the question of the A-type and B-type personality, critics remind us that most people do not fall into these clear-cut categories. Certainly there are people at both extremes of the spectrum. There are some people who are obvious A types, and others who are obvious B types, just as there are obvious introverts and extroverts. However, the number who are in either of the extreme groups is a small proportion of the whole. This makes the entire concept open to debate. Nearly all the evidence for linking A-type personalities with heart disease is in the popular literature.

### Current medical views

Although doctors are still arguing about stress, the term, perhaps significantly, is cropping up far more frequently in textbooks and medical papers than ever before. A search on the word "stress" in any medical database will turn up thousands of examples. This is partly because the word has become so fashionable that it is used in all kinds of contexts and with a range of meanings.

Many diseases are now believed to have at least some basis in stress. Typical is the state of opinion on stress and peptic ulceration of the lining of the stomach and the first part of the small intestine (see Duodenum). Most of the research into this question has been in the form of retrospective studies looking back to see whether people with peptic ulceration were people who had been stressed. This is not considered the ideal method, and too much is left to the opinion of either the patient or the doctor.

Prospective studies to see whether stressed people later develop ulcers are better. One 13-year prospective study of over 4,000 people with no history of ulcers showed that those who were aware of stress in their lives were more likely to develop peptic ulcers than those who were not. Again, however, the assessment of stress has to be subjective, and this makes convincing research difficult to organize. Only objective evidence is fully acceptable to science. One study, however, found many more personality disturbances in people with peptic ulcers than in those with kidney stones or gallstones. Currently it is agreed that more prospective studies are needed to determine the role of emotional stress in peptic ulceration.

These doubts have not prevented many scientific doctors from trying to produce theories to explain the relationship between stress and the processes that lead to disease. New models of how stress might operate appear regularly in the medical and psychological journals. A review of the medical literature indicates some support for the opinion that stress operates on the immune system. There is an awareness of the link between the immune system and brain processes concerned with thought, environmental perception, behavior, appreciation of stress, and so on. The immune system does not work in isolation in its defense against infection, tumors, and foreign material (see Immune System). A new branch of medical science, called psychoneuroimmunology, is concerned with the study of interactions between the mind and the immune system (see Mind).

## Psychoneuroimmunology

Doctors are now gaining a clearer understanding of the ways in which hormones can affect the immune system. They are also discovering that immune system regulation can be mediated by direct nerve connections to the lymphoid tissue of the system (see Lymphatic System). These advances begin to explain much that was previously obscure about the way in which the body can respond to stress. This research also promises to advance people's understanding of how human behavior can control the function of the immune system and how psychosocial factors and emotional states can affect the development of diseases such as infections and cancers (see Cancer; Infection and Infectious Diseases).

The science of psychoneuroimmunology is still in its infancy, but remarkable advances in our knowledge of both neurologic and immunologic control mechanisms are making it increasingly clear that there are previously unsuspected ways in which stress can cause various diseases (see Nervous System; Neurology and Neurosurgery).

## Post-traumatic stress disorder

For those who respond badly to stress, there are certain warning signs suggesting danger. These include increasing irritability, loss of appetite, sleeping difficulties, loss of concentration, greater difficulty

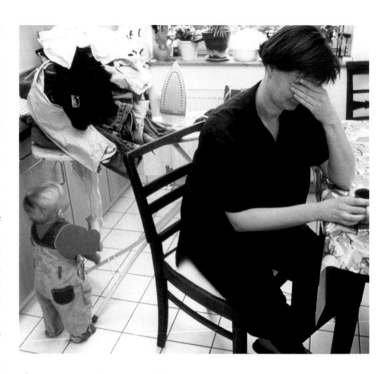

▲ *Some people find child rearing particularly stressful. The anxiety and worry of keeping a young child in good health and away from danger can take its toll of stress on a parent.*

in making decisions, inability to relax, short fuse, and anger over trivial matters. All these are commonplace.

Less common is the acute stress reaction which relates obviously to a particular event, and which is followed within about an hour by obvious symptoms. These may include anger, despair, aggression, withdrawal, or excessive grief. The outlook in this condition is good, but time is required for recovery. No one would try to deny that there are levels of stress so severe that many people exposed to them would suffer psychological damage. Again, the outcome in such cases varies with the personality. When people are involved in major disasters, such as train or plane crashes or earthquakes, many come through the experience apparently unharmed; others react very badly.

In World War I, soldiers were exposed to appalling stress from long periods of intense artillery or mortar bombardment and small arms fire. These unfortunates were frequently required to get up out of their trenches and run across open terrain in the face of machine gun fire and almost certain death. Those who broke down were said to suffer from lack of moral fiber. Those who ran away were tried for cowardice and shot. Thousands who survived these ordeals subsequently suffered from what was then called shell shock, and what is now called post-traumatic stress disorder.

This disorder features a repetitive reliving of the stressful event or events, with intrusive flashback memories and nightmares. Any event or circumstance that reminds the sufferer of the stressor event causes serious distress. The features of stress listed above are often present, and there may be loss of memory (amnesia) of the event. If not treated, the disorder can become permanent.

See also: Adrenal glands; Anxiety; Blood pressure; Colon and colitis; Exercise; Heart attack; Post-traumatic stress disorder; Psychosomatic problems; Relaxation; Ulcers

# Stress management

**Everyone is subject to stress at some time, but it can take a serious toll on general health if it is ignored or tackled in the wrong way. Recognizing the need to deal with stress is the first step to successful stress management.**

**My job is mentally demanding and I often stay late. I get a lot of satisfaction from doing it well. Is stress always such a bad thing?**

Individuals vary in their ability to cope with stress and you evidently thrive on some pressure, seeing it as an opportunity to achieve. However, make sure that the demands of your job don't throw your life off balance; make sure you're eating well, relaxing, and having a social life. Make time for leisure pursuits and exercise to throw off the tensions of the day.

**Over the last few years I've had many problems, and broken up a long-term relationship. My mother thinks I'll feel better if I tell her about it, but I find it hard to talk about it. Is there any harm in keeping my feelings to myself?**

Showing a brave face isn't a good way of dealing with stress. Most people find it helps to air their emotions so that they can grieve for a loss such as yours, or put their fears into perspective. Don't talk to your mother if you don't want to, but consider talking to a friend or a counselor. Or you could write your thoughts and feelings in a journal or in a letter that you may or may not send.

**I work and when I get home, my husband expects me to do all the chores. I'm stressed and tired. Are there any quick relaxation techniques that will help?**

You could take 10 or 20 minutes a day to focus on slowing your breathing and relaxing all your muscles. However, you could also ease your stress by changing your lifestyle. Discuss your workload with your supervisor and also with your husband. Assertiveness training might help you gain the confidence to refuse to take on more work than you can easily cope with.

When someone is subject to pressures or tensions, his or her body reacts by triggering the production of various chemicals or hormones, such as epinephrine, that prepare for flight from danger or fighting back against attack. The heart rate speeds up, boosting the blood supply to the muscles; glucose and fats flood into the bloodstream to supply extra energy; blood pressure rises; and blood flow is diverted away from the intestinal tract to more immediately useful areas. In complex modern societies, there is little place for this kind of reaction, since it is often counterproductive. If the body regularly experiences this physiological reaction to stress without any outlet, the result may in some cases be a stress-related illness, from tension headache or backache to serious or even fatal illness. Prolonged stress is known to play a role in heart disease and high blood pressure, which can lead to stroke. Psychological problems resulting from stress include irritation, anxiety, and exhaustion, and severe emotional stress can contribute to mental breakdown. Stress may also be a significant factor in encouraging smoking, heavy drinking, and drug abuse, all of which produce ill effects. Successful stress management aims to avoid these consequences by teaching people the best strategies for responding to pressures.

## Recognizing and facing up to stress

Certain situations are high in the stress ratings: for example, life-changing events such as bereavement, job loss, relationship breakup, and even positive events such as getting married or moving house. The event, however, is less important than the individual's perception of it—for example, a change of job may be disrupting for one person but a pleasant change for another. Personality matters too; some people naturally take setbacks in their stride or see a problem as a challenge, while others tend to become very anxious or depressed (see Depression).

Stress, however, is not a force outside people's control, although this may be the feeling of those suffering from it. Keeping a stress diary for a few weeks is one way to assess the amount of stress and its source: people set aside a few minutes at the end of each day to describe when they were tense or upset, or events that made them feel anxious, noting their reaction and how they should have dealt with the event. A pattern may well emerge, showing that most stress

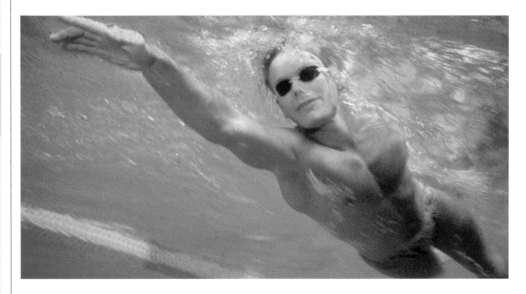

▲ *A hectic lifestyle makes a certain amount of stress unavoidable. Positive steps to ease tension are taking exercise such as swimming, or other sports.*

comes from work overload or from difficulties with personal relationships. This knowledge can be used to help develop an action plan that will help people regain control and draw on strategies to tackle stress produced by different problems.

## Time and energy management

If stress seems overwhelming, people should review their life and what they want from relationships, and work. The time and energy allocated to each area of their life should be balanced. Some people work too hard at the expense of their personal life; strategies to deal with this include setting goals, such as gaining a better job or learning to say no to a friend's demands; and prioritizing tasks in order of their importance. A time-management strategy that allows more time to spend on enjoyable or important activities encourages a sense of achievement and control.

### Stress: How well do you cope?

Natural reactions to any stressful situation may be positive or potentially damaging. Adaptive or positive tactics are those that help you face the problem causing the stress, and so find a solution. These tactics include:

Expressing emotions, whether sadness or anger

Talking over the problem with friends

Thinking through the problem to try to understand it

Seeking support from others

Setting priorities for tackling problems

Acting to solve a problem

Negative tactics involve avoiding the issue and may enable someone to cope in the short term, but over time will aggravate the stress. These tactics include:

Bottling up emotions

Avoiding other people

Worrying

Losing sleep

Eating more or not eating

Fantasizing about outcomes without taking any action

Keeping busy or finding distractions

Drinking or smoking more, or resorting to drugs

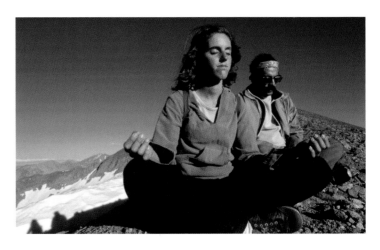

▲ *Meditation, particularly outdoors, is one way of helping to alleviate the stresses and tensions of everyday life.*

Assertiveness training helps counter stress caused by overwork or conflicting demands at work and home. Nonassertive people find it hard to refuse others' demands and to express their own needs, laying themselves open to stress at work or in personal relationships. It is possible to learn assertive behavior skills—this is different from behaving aggressively—from self-help books or organized programs.

Another approach to dealing with stress is to try to change the way stressful experiences are perceived, a process sometimes called cognitive reappraisal. Some people respond to distressing events in a negative way, but if negative thoughts and worries are recognized as such, tactics can be developed to resist them, such as steering thoughts to a more enjoyable and positive area.

## Relaxation and support

Relaxation techniques help to counter the effects of stress. Various methods have been developed, involving exercises such as tensing and then relaxing muscles, visualizing a peaceful place, and concentrating on breathing slowly and deeply. Learning to pause and relax for a few seconds before tackling a stressful situation is a useful technique. More formal methods of relaxation include autogenic training, or self-hypnosis, and meditation, both of which require training by an instructor or therapist. Transcendental meditation (TM) has been shown to reduce anxiety and improve performance, as well as having long-term benefits in the treatment of high blood pressure and other stress-related diseases.

Leisure activities are helpful, and physical exercise is a good counter to stress. Research shows that aerobic exercise such as swimming, running, cycling, or dancing can improve people's psychological ability to deal with stress, reduce depression, and aid sleeping, and competitive sports provide a way to relieve frustration. Poor nutrition, with a high intake of sugary, fatty, and processed foods, can reduce resistance to stress, and using caffeine and high-sugar snacks will sap energy levels. Eating a balanced diet will provide more energy to cope with stress. Sharing feelings with friends, coworkers, or family is useful; bottling up emotions is rarely helpful. However, being able to turn to others for social activities is valuable. Those without social support networks tend to be more prone to stress-related disease and depression.

*See also:* **Meditation; Nutrition**

# Stretch marks

**Anyone can develop stretch marks, and many women frequently do in pregnancy. There is some doubt, however, that skin stretching is the principal cause of these permanent marks, and that they can be prevented.**

Human skin is naturally elastic, and can normally stretch considerably to accommodate a sudden change in weight or in the shape of the mass that it covers. The tissue beneath the skin surface develops as we grow so that the skin area above it gradually increases. If very rapid physical expansion takes place, the elastic tissue may be put under intolerable strain. It is not certain, however, that stretch marks are simply just a matter of skin stretching. They are certainly common in pregancy but much less common in obesity. Some experts believe that they probably result from the increased levels of free cortisol present in pregnancy.

The medical term "stria" means a "stripe" and does not imply a causal factor such as stretching. Striae are a feature of many medical conditions, especially Cushing's syndrome in which abnormal quantities of adrenal cortisol are produced. Striae may also occur in people, especially women, who are given large doses of steroids for medical purposes. Striae are a feature of Marfan's syndrome, the nephrotic syndrome, and the disease lichen planus.

The redness of a stretch mark fades in a matter of months, but the skin surface never returns to its previous condition. A papery kind of scar tissue will remain, and the stretch marks will look like pale or silvery threadlike lines (see Scars).

## When stretch marks occur

Stretch marks can occur during puberty (see Adolescence; Puberty). As the hormonal balance changes, teenage girls may quickly put on weight in specific areas. The sites most likely to be affected are the breasts, hips, thighs, and buttocks. Stretch marks may be more likely to occur in girls who are already slightly overweight, although they can affect girls who have developed large breasts at a particularly fast rate during puberty.

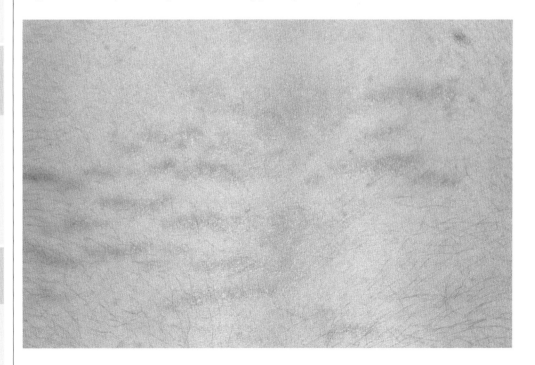

▲ *Stretch marks on the back of a teenage boy who had been overweight. Stretch marks (shiny streaks that appear on the skin) most commonly appear in adolescent girls and in women during pregnancy, but can occur as the result of any sudden weight gain.*

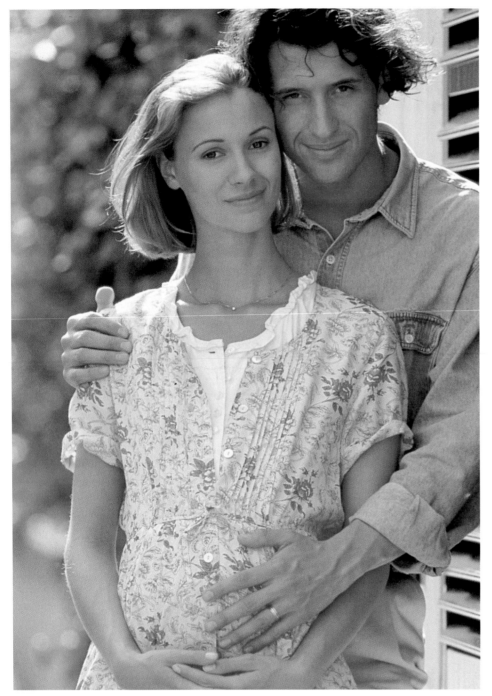

▲ *Pregnant women often find that stretch marks appear on their breasts and abdomen. Generally they will find that the marks fade quite rapidly after the birth.*

## Can stretch marks be prevented?

Since the actual cause of stretch marks remains uncertain and since clinical experience has shown it to be unpredictable who will develop stretch marks and, if so, how severe they will be, it is difficult to say if stretch marks can be prevented. All that can be done is to act on the assumption that one possible factor may be the rate at which the skin is stretched.

Women who are careful about what they eat and how much weight they put on during pregnancy may be less likely to develop stretch marks than those who tend to eat to excess. Even though stretch marks on the breasts and abdomen may be inevitable, those on other areas of the body (the legs, arms, hips, and thighs) are probably the result of being overweight. There is no evidence that one type of skin is more prone to stretch marks than another.

If a woman is developing stretch marks during pregnancy she should immediately review her diet. As a result of hormonal changes calories are burned less efficiently than before the pregnancy, so to compensate for this she may have to eat less fat and carbohydrates (see Diet). Her doctor or prenatal clinic will be able to advise her on what her weight should be during pregnancy, and help her to plan her diet accordingly. Some stretch marks are unavoidable, but early preventive action may minimize the possibility of getting more marks later in the pregnancy.

Some people maintain that oils or creams rubbed into the skin of the breasts and abdomen will prevent stretch marks, but most doctors will point out that no amount of lubrication of the skin surface affects the changes beneath it. However, many women find that the skin becomes dry and flaky during pregnancy and that an oil or cream helps considerably with this problem. There is certainly no harm in using such products, and if a pregnant woman takes care of herself in this way she will also quickly become aware of unnecessary weight gain and so be more careful about eating too much during pregnancy.

Stretch marks are likely to be worse in women who are carrying twins because the abdomen will be stretched far more than it would be in a single pregnancy.

Extreme fluid retention or an excess of amniotic fluid can also result in particularly severe stretch marks. In these cases plastic surgery may be advised after pregnancy, but this is unusual for most women (see Plastic and Reconstructive Surgery).

Stretch marks will remain a reddish color throughout a pregnancy, but will usually gradually lose their color in the months after the baby has been born. Some marks may hardly show after a few months, but others will be visible indefinitely. Affected skin can also be shinier and thinner than the surrounding skin and may become less elastic. In some cases, stretch marks may be so severe that they resemble surgical scars, such as the abdominal scar left by an appendectomy.

Prolonged treatment with steroid drugs can also cause stretch marks, and there will also be weight gain from taking large doses of steroid drugs (see Steroids).

**See also: Skin and skin diseases**

# Stroke

**With little or no warning a stroke can cause sudden weakness, paralysis, or even death. Nevertheless, however fearsome this common affliction may be, rehabilitation can help survivors overcome any resulting disability.**

## Questions and Answers

**My mother had a serious stroke when she was 53. Does this put me at risk of having one too?**

Not necessarily. Your chances of having a stroke depend to some extent on what caused your mother's disease. If high blood pressure was the cause, then it may be advisable to have your blood pressure checked so that, if high blood pressure is found, suitable treatment can be given. If there is a long history of strokes in your family, then it is important that you do not add to the risk by smoking.

**Does taking the Pill increase the risk of having a stroke?**

In a tiny number of women, strokes have occurred while they were on the Pill. For this reason doctors try to discourage women who are over 40 from taking the Pill. There is far less risk in women who are under 40. However, doctors will try to dissuade women under 40 from continuing with the Pill if they have a history of migraine, as it does slightly increase the chances of having a stroke at a younger age.

**Is there any surgery that can treat people who have had a stroke?**

Strokes from leaking berry aneurysms can sometimes be treated surgically to stop the bleeding and prevent further hemorrhage. Occasionally, one of the larger arteries in the neck may be narrowed or roughened inside, and surgery to correct this may prevent further damaging strokes.

**My father has just had a stroke and can't speak. Will his speech return?**

Yes, it is very likely that his ability to speak will come back, at least to some extent. Sometimes people are not able to speak at all in the first few days after a stroke, but later recover almost completely.

Strokes often (though not exclusively) attack older people and are one of the most common causes of death throughout the Western world. However, present advances in medical research, particularly in connection with the role of high blood pressure, have helped doctors' understanding of this illness. Many strokes are now preventable through early identification and treatment of those at risk.

### What is a stroke?

Most people have some idea of what a stroke is; such knowledge is a testament to how often the disease occurs. The common factor in all strokes is that, owing to a disease of the blood vessel that supplies a particular part of the brain, a section of the brain suddenly stops working. The person involved often has little or no warning that something is wrong before he or she is struck down, most often with weakness or paralysis down one side of the body. This condition may be accompanied by aphasia (loss of speech) or by other problems in higher brain functions. A small number of strokes occur in parts of the brain that do not control the body's movement, so that paralysis does not occur (see Brain).

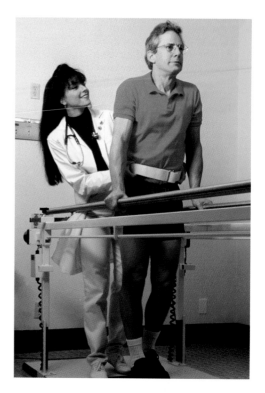

▲ *A stroke need not signal the end to a person's active life. With physical therapy, it is often possible to restore the function of affected limbs to varying degrees.*

### What causes a stroke?

Like the rest of the body, the brain must have a constant supply of blood reaching it through its arteries. If one of these arteries becomes blocked, the part of the brain that it feeds will die because of the lack of oxygen. There are many cross-connections in the brain between neighboring blood vessels, so that the area of damage is generally restricted. However, even the part of the brain that does not die may swell and damage the rest of the brain. The other way in which strokes may be caused is that blood vessels in the brain burst. When this happens, the blood rushes into the brain under pressure, severely damaging nerve fibers (see Nervous System).

These two basic mechanisms, cerebral infarction (when the artery is blocked) and cerebral hemorrhage (when there is bleeding into the brain), can be brought about by a variety of disorders.

Obstruction of an artery in the brain can result from a disease that produces a blockage in the artery itself (a cerebral thrombosis), or when a blood clot passes up the blood supply to the brain artery and gets stuck there. This is called a cerebral embolism.

Thrombosis (or blood clotting) generally occurs when an artery of the brain becomes narrowed: fatty material accumulates in the walls of the artery. This is what happens in the disease called atherosclerosis, which also causes the heart's blood vessels to clot, resulting in heart attacks (see Heart Attack). Occasionally, other problems in the arteries can cause thrombosis. These include inflammation of the artery, which can occur on its own or as a result of some serious infections.

Embolisms can be caused by heart diseases or by disorders in the main arteries in the neck from which the blood enters the brain. Heart disease and strokes are thus linked, not only

## Questions and Answers

**Does everyone who has had a stroke have to be hospitalized?**

This would depend on the severity of the stroke, and whether or not the facilities available in the stroke patient's home enable him or her to be properly looked after. In some areas, special teams of physical therapists are available to treat people in their own homes. However, people with strokes often need to remain in the hospital while they are very disabled so that their stroke can be properly assessed, in terms of treatment and of prevention of further strokes.

**Is there any point in having someone's blood pressure treated after a stroke, or is this like shutting the stable door after the horse has bolted?**

Immediately after a stroke, the blood pressure is usually left alone for a few days, since a sudden drop may impair the flow of blood to the damaged areas in the brain. However, careful studies have shown that it is important to treat the blood pressure vigorously to prevent further strokes, which might cause further disability.

**My uncle had a bad heart attack and a few weeks later had a stroke that paralyzed his left side. Was this connected with his heart attack, and why did this happen?**

After a heart attack, blood clots may form on the inside wall of the chamber of the heart. Occasionally, part of a clot can become dislodged and fly upward to block off one of the brain's blood vessels, thus producing a stroke. Patients who have had very serious heart attacks can be given anticoagulant drugs to help prevent this.

**Is it possible to prevent strokes?**

Yes, in some cases. If patients who have high blood pressure are identified and treated early, this can greatly reduce the risk of a stroke.

because the same disease of the arteries can cause trouble in both the heart and the brain, but also because in many diseases of the heart, blood clots form on the valves or on the damaged inside walls of the heart and these then fly off as emboli (see Heart Disease).

Cerebral hemorrhages (in which the blood vessels in the brain burst) also have a number of causes (see Hemorrhage). The most common cause is that there are weak places (called aneurysms) in the walls of the brain's arteries which then burst, often because they have been weakened by atherosclerosis. In the larger brain arteries at the base of the skull these aneurysms may be congenital, though they may not rupture until late in life, if at all. Less common causes of cerebral hemorrhage can occur as a result of the presence of small, abnormally formed blood vessels in the brain, rather like the strawberry marks that are a similar abnormality of the blood vessels in the skin. This is called arteriovenous anomaly, and again this condition is congenital.

### Who is at risk?

Certain people have a higher risk of having strokes than others. The main conditions that predispose a person toward a stroke are atherosclerosis, high blood pressure, having high serum

**DAMAGE CAUSED BY A STROKE**

loss of feeling and strength

disturbance in reading ability and sight; possible difficulties with speech and swallowing

anterior cerebral artery

middle cerebral artery

posterior cerebral artery

circle of Willis

ophthalmic arteries

disturbance in sight and speech

basilar artery

internal carotid arteries

circle of Willis

vertebral arteries

disturbance of vital brain stem functions such as respiration, often with sudden death

middle cerebral arteries

anterior cerebral arteries

posterior cerebral arteries

basilar artery

physical disability, particularly in face and arm

vertebral arteries

possible loss of feeling and strength

internal carotid arteries

▲ A stroke can be caused by a blockage in any of the four pairs of cerebral arteries. Each type has different results, depending on the area of the brain that is affected. A blockage in an anterior artery is common, and one in the basilar is usually fatal.

## MAJOR CAUSES OF STROKES

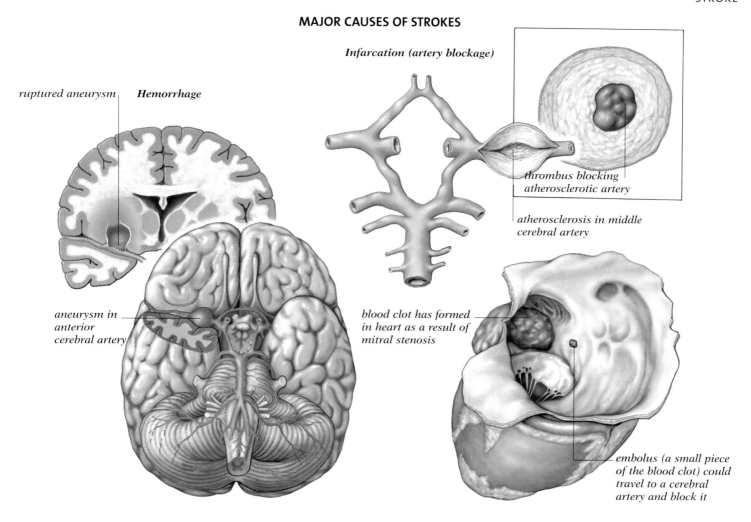

*Infarction (artery blockage)*

ruptured aneurysm | **Hemorrhage**

thrombus blocking
atherosclerotic artery

atherosclerosis in middle
cerebral artery

aneurysm in
anterior
cerebral artery

blood clot has formed
in heart as a result of
mitral stenosis

embolus (a small piece
of the blood clot) could
travel to a cerebral
artery and block it

▲ *Strokes can be caused by hemorrhages or blockages (infarctions) in the brain. Many hemorrhages are caused by the rupturing of weakened arteries (aneurysms). Infarctions are caused either when a blood clot forms in a diseased cerebral artery (thrombus), or when a clot travels from another area of the body, such as the damaged walls of the heart, and lodges in the brain (embolus).*

cholesterol, having diabetes, and smoking cigarettes (see Cholesterol). In addition, strokes seem to run in some families, though because the condition is so common, this is difficult to prove. Finally, there are people with heart diseases that can cause a stroke by embolism. Therefore, people with a high risk can often be identified, and preventive measures can be taken to reduce the chances of a stroke.

### Symptoms

Many stroke patients have a warning attack in the weeks or months before a major stroke. These warning attacks take the form of short-lived episodes of weakness down one side, or transient blacking out of vision in one eye—a sign of blockage in one of the blood vessels to the retina. These warnings are called transient ischemic attacks (TIAs) and they must never be ignored. Medical attention at the stage of the TIA can save life. In most cases, disabilities such as loss of function on one side of the body or loss of speech reach their maximum within minutes, though occasionally it may take hours. In the following days and weeks, there will be an improvement as some

of the brain cells recover. After six months the disabilities will be considerably less than they were at the onset of the stroke.

Other symptoms may include loss of vision in the right- or left-hand half of the visual field of both eyes, difficulty in dressing or finding the way around familiar surroundings, and various other subtle difficulties in brain function. If a large area of the brain was damaged at the start of the stroke, the patient may not have a clear awareness of what has happened, or may ignore everything that happens on one side of his or her body. As the damaged brain swells, he or she may become drowsy or lose consciousness (see Unconsciousness). This may happen much more quickly in brain hemorrhages, since the surge of blood into the brain causes damage to the mechanisms that maintain alertness.

### Treatment

Initial treatment consists of limiting the amount of damage that may be caused by swelling spreading to the unaffected parts of the brain. This is done by paying close attention to the blood pressure and administering certain drugs, particularly steroids. Very seldom can surgeons remove the blood clots that are causing pressure, since they are often situated in inaccessible parts of the brain.

However, the main care of patients who have had strokes lies in the hands of the nursing staff, physical therapists, speech therapists, and occupational therapists. Careful nursing is very important to prevent the emergence of bedsores and chest troubles, which can seriously impair a patient's recovery from a stroke (see Bedsores). During this vulnerable period when the stroke patient is often

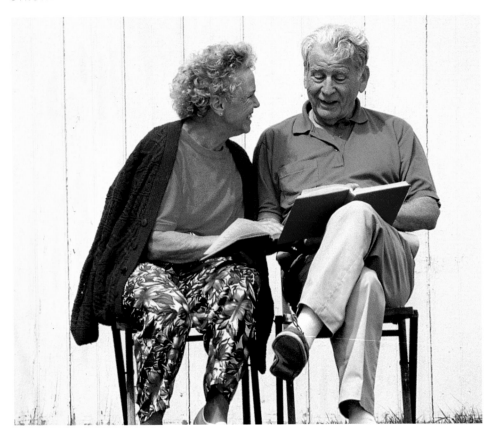

▲ *One of the most important stages in the recovery of a stroke patient takes place at home, where the support of family and friends becomes vital.*

▼ *Communication boards are available for stroke victims with speech impairment. This patient can point to words and illustrations that express his thoughts or needs.*

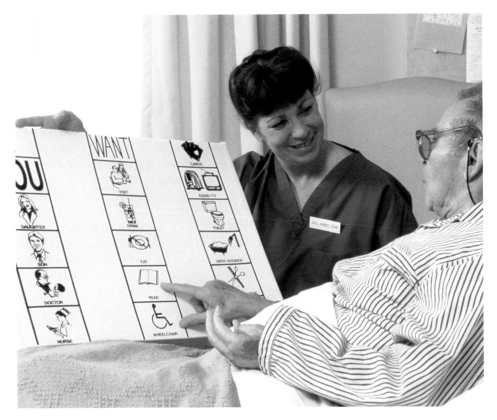

unable to undertake his or her own care, good nursing can literally save a life.

Physical therapists maximize the effect of movement as it returns to affected limbs. Later they become even more vital because the therapy they suggest may make the difference between a patient's becoming seriously disabled or able to fend for himself or herself despite residual disabilities.

Treatment is in two stages. First, physical therapists ensure that the unused limbs remain supple and that unnecessary stiffness does not set in. Later, when the patient is ambulant (and this happens early, since prolonged periods in bed can be dangerous), the physical therapist concentrates on overcoming the abnormal reflex movements that interfere with the return of more useful muscle power (see Reflexes).

Speech therapy plays an important role when the stroke has affected the power of speech. Speech therapists will be able to identify the difficulties the patient has and will work to encourage the return of speech, which often does happen to a greater or lesser extent. Further treatment by speech therapists consists of retraining patients with aphasia to make the best of the speech faculties that are left (see Speech).

Occupational therapists try to prepare the patient for a return to as normal a life as possible. The therapist assesses the patient, and works out ways of overcoming problems that resist physical therapy.

## The stroke patient at home

Many stroke patients are hospitalized while they are physically dependent (often in special stroke units), and then further recovery can be looked for when they go home. The patient's family will need a lot of support and guidance to make sure that they are not so overprotective that they slow his or her recovery. Therefore, the work of the physical and occupational therapists often extends to the home, where they can continue to supervise the patient's recovery. Special aids are available for facilitating such everyday tasks as taking a shower, cooking, and eating, which often present difficulties.

## Preventing a stroke

The recent advances in stroke research have been concerned with prevention. The fact that in recent years in the United States the number of strokes has declined is indicative of the effectiveness of the research. This is due to the recognition of the importance of

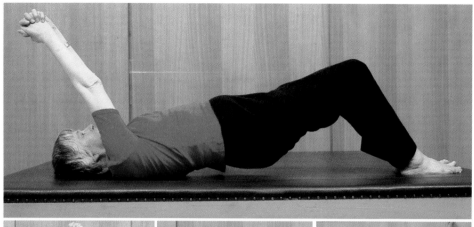

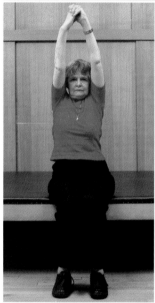
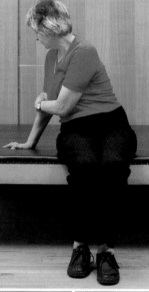
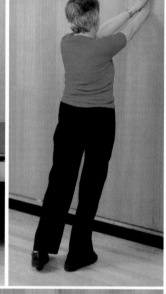

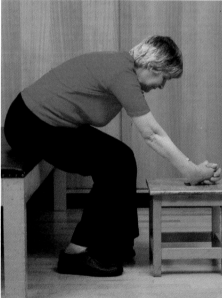
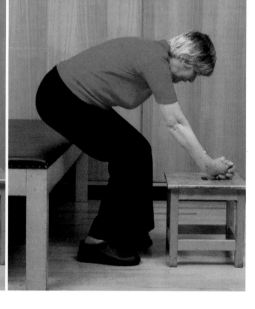

▲ *Stroke patients can exercise in their own homes. Exercises include using the strong arm to support the weak arm (top left) or paralyzed side (top right) by pulling it up. Additional strengthening can be achieved by doing swiveling (middle left) or pressing exercises (middle right), which require propping up the weak arm. Better balance can be gained by raising the body to a half-sitting position (above).*

transient ischemic attacks (TIAs) and the identification and treatment of high blood pressure. TIAs cause temporary failure of part of the brain, owing to reduced blood supply. They often herald a stroke; awareness of this has provided doctors with the opportunity for positive intervention to avoid strokes.

Most people with high blood pressure feel well and may need convincing to take their pills regularly to keep it down. Generally, the doctor will take the blood pressure as a matter of routine when they consult him or her and will be able to detect high blood pressure before it leads to trouble.

After minor strokes from which the patient may have recovered, it is an important part of treatment to try to prevent another more serious episode from occurring. Surgery can sometimes be performed on the large blood vessels in the neck. This may be done if the blood vessels have roughened parts in their lining from which clots fly off as emboli.

Small doses of aspirin are also being tried for stroke prevention. It has been found that small amounts of the drug can affect the clotting ability of the blood to a degree sufficient to prevent the brain's blood vessels from becoming obstructed (see Aspirin and Analgesics). Anticoagulant drugs reduce the blood's liability to clot, and these are used to prevent a stroke when one of the predisposing heart conditions is identified. Many other drugs that can prevent a stroke in those at risk are now undergoing trials.

## Outlook

Although a stroke can be fatal, most victims recover to some degree. At least half of those who have had a stroke progress to a point where they can look after themselves, and most people paralyzed by strokes learn to walk again. Only about 5 percent of patients require long-term institutional care. While the remainder of stroke sufferers may have to depend on relatives to look after them at home, they or their caregivers should make full use of the variety of home aids and of the hospital and therapeutic treatments available to them to help patients overcome or live with their disabilities.

*See also:* Aphasia; Arteries and artery disease; Blood pressure; Brain damage and disease; Paralysis; Physical therapy; Rehabilitation; Speech therapy; Thrombosis; Transient ischemic attack

# Sty

## Questions and Answers

**Are sties caused by dandruff?**

Sties do occur more commonly in people suffering from seborrheic dermatitis. This condition affects the scalp and produces dandruff, and causes a scaly inflammation of the eyebrows and eyelids. When the dandruff is treated the sties often clear up too.

**I have heard that sties are very infectious. Is this true?**

The bacteria causing sties are infectious and certain virulent types seem to be responsible for recurrent infections. Anyone with a sty should avoid rubbing the eyes; this can spread the infection to other sebaceous glands. A separate towel and washcloth should be used to prevent spreading the infection. An antibiotic ointment may prevent the discharging pus from infecting other glands.

**Is it safe to pull out the eyelash in a sty?**

Yes, the pus will then drain out. Soften the eyelid with a hot compress to reduce the pain. The eyelash can be pulled out with a pair of tweezers and the sty should discharge spontaneously. If the relevant eyelash is not obvious, the eyelids should be left alone. Either the sty is not yet ripe or it may be an internal cyst, in which case there is no eyelash to remove.

**I have a small, painless nodule under my eyelid. Is this a sty?**

It may be a meibomian cyst. Although sometimes called an internal sty, it is not a sty or an infection but an accumulation of trapped gland secretion. It is felt as a hard lump like a small hailstone. There is no need to do anything, but it can be removed surgically for cosmetic reasons.

**Children and adolescents often suffer from sties—painful and unsightly swellings of the eyelid. While minor surgery may be required in some cases, antibiotic ointment and first aid are usually all that is needed.**

Two different types of eyelid glands can become infected. On the outside are sebaceous glands associated with the eyelashes, which secrete greasy sebum to protect the surface of the eye (see Sebaceous Glands). However, this sebum may block the gland and trap bacteria, and an external sty will then result. On the inside the eye has a further special line of glands called the meibomian glands. These are also sebaceous glands, but have no associated hair follicles. They open through the conjunctiva to the back of the eyelid and the secretion they produce may also block the gland. This is called a meibomian cyst. Some meibomian cysts become infected and form small abcesses, but these should be distinguished from a regular sty.

## Causes
Sties are associated with a general tendency to dry skin and eczema, as in seborrheic dermatitis (see Dermatitis; Eczema). Dandruff and flaking skin around the eyelashes and eyebrows are related to this condition, and sties may be a complication of it. However, many children get sties with no underlying skin disease, and in these cases the cause is unknown. If sties recur, an underlying condition must be suspected. As in all infections, ill health and lack of physical fitness will make sties more common.

## Symptoms
The eye may feel uncomfortable for a day or so before the sty appears; itchiness and a sensation of a foreign body in the eye may be felt. The sty appears over the course of one to two days, starting as a local painful spot and then swelling to a red, angry pustule. An external sty is easily recognized on the eyelid, but to see a meibomian gland infection, the eyelid must be turned out to expose the back. Meibomian abcesses are usually more painful than external ones, since the distending meibomian gland will stretch the whole eyelid.

As a sty forms, the pain in the lid and the feeling of grittiness get worse. Bright light aggravates the pain (photophobia) and the eye seems to be continually weeping. A fretful child

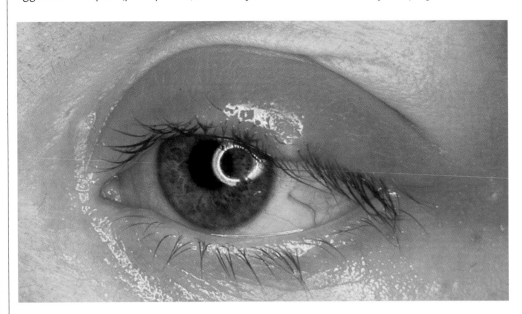

▲ *Infection of one of the sebaceous glands in the eyelid can produce an external sty— an obvious red, angry pustule (above) that causes pain, and a feeling of grittiness.*

## If you have a sty

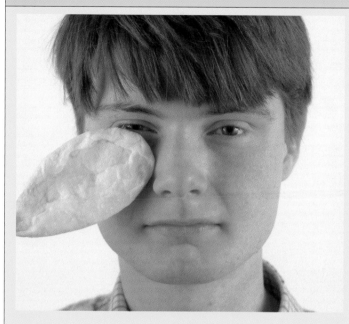

**Do**

Do take steps to control dandruff. Wash hair regularly with an antidandruff shampoo to prevent recurrence.

Do apply a hot compress—a wooden spoon wrapped in a washcloth held under hot water will suffice. Hold to the eye for 10-minute periods to relieve pain and inflammation.

Do remove the offending eyelash if the sty is external; it will then discharge.

**Do not**

Do not rub the eye, however tempting rubbing may be, as it risks spreading the infection to other sebaceous glands.

Do not share a towel or washcloth.

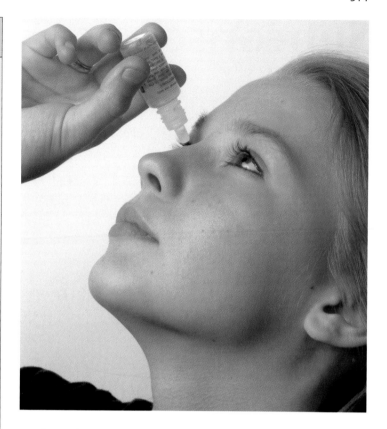

▲ *If sties keep recurring, a course of antibiotic eyedrops may help to prevent any discharging pus from infecting other sebaceous glands in the eyelid.*

with photophobia, a runny nose from crying, and eye problems may be diagnosed as having a more serious illness such as measles; but detection of a sty and the absence of symptoms in the other eye should clarify the problem.

### Treatment

If an incipient sty is recognized early enough, antibiotic eye ointment or drops can prevent the sty from forming. However, it is much more common to find that by the time a diagnosis has been made, the pustule is already formed, and antibiotics are then ineffective. The only treatment at this stage is to encourage the pus to discharge.

Local warmth from a hot compress will increase the blood flow and soften the eyelid, relieving pain, and encouraging the infection to clear. A simple hot compress can be made by using a clean washcloth wound on a wooden spoon and held under the hot faucet. It should be as warm as can be tolerated and held in contact with the closed eye for 10 minutes at a time. For an external sty, the offending hair follicle can easily be identified. If the eyelash is pulled out with tweezers the sty will often discharge spontaneously, relieving the pain and the swelling.

Meibomain abcesses are more difficult to deal with. The infected meibomian gland tries in vain to discharge to the surface, but the tough eyelid prevents this. The result is that the white cells eventually overcome the infection—so the symptoms go away—but they remain in situ as a cyst of sterile pus. This can be felt as a little painless nodule under the eyelid, and a small surgical operation is required to remove it. Under local anesthesia the eyelid is turned back and the cyst incised; the pus discharges and the conjunctival surface swiftly heals.

With recurrent sties, antibiotic ointments may be helpful in preventing discharging pus from infecting other sebaceous glands on the eyelid. Rubbing the eye should be avoided, as this can transfer the infection; and controlling dandruff is also important, since this condition seems to cause sties. When inflammation of the eyelids (blepharitis) is the cause, a prolonged course of antibiotics in conjunction with mild steroid drops may be helpful.

Some children suffer from multiple recurrent sties. They do not harm the eye but they are painful and unpleasant. The cause is still unknown in most cases, but the problem should be discussed with a doctor, since there may be an underlying problem, such as seborrheic dermatitis, which will respond to treatment.

*See also:* **Dandruff; Pain; Pus**

# Subconscious

**Are dreams from the subconscious?**

No one knows where dreams come from. They are the result of some kind of mental activity and occur when the brain is in a state of arousal that brings about bodily effects including rapid eye movements. Dreams are often related to anxiety. The general view is that they are an attempt by the mind to make sense of material that is not sufficiently organized into a unified whole to be effectively stored in memory.

**Do artistic people have very active subconscious minds?**

Yes. Artistic creativity is largely a matter of subconscious activity, although, to be effective, the artist must engage in a hard conscious work. Literary artists are constantly surprised at what their subconscious minds produce. It seems that much of creativity consists of a subconscious synthesis of ideas and data.

**I want to have psychotherapy, but worry about what is in my subconscious. Should I go ahead?**

With a psychotherapist you respect and trust, you will find that he or she will support you through the journey of self-discovery. You may find that the more you understand about yourself, the stronger and less fearful you will feel.

**If I do something my sister dislikes, she says I subconsciously resent her. Is she right?**

Your sister may be right or wrong, but such an observation is not, by itself, helpful. It is used merely as a weapon in an argument. Explain that you can sort out your feelings only if you trust one another enough to talk about them without such accusations.

**The subconscious is a part of the mind where our deepest fears, childhood experiences, and primitive memories are stored. The store of information is often outside conscious awareness, but it can be brought into consciousness.**

Human behavior is largely conditioned by past experience, beliefs, and feelings of which people are usually very much aware. Sometimes, however, people's actions may seem out of character, and although they felt that these actions were perfectly reasonable actions at the time, subsequently they find it difficult to explain why they acted as they did. This is just one piece of evidence for the existence of the subconscious mind.

There is other evidence: for example, people often hear their name mentioned in a conversation, even if they were not listening for it and could not hear anything else that was being said; or they will frequently notice a clock has stopped ticking, even though they were

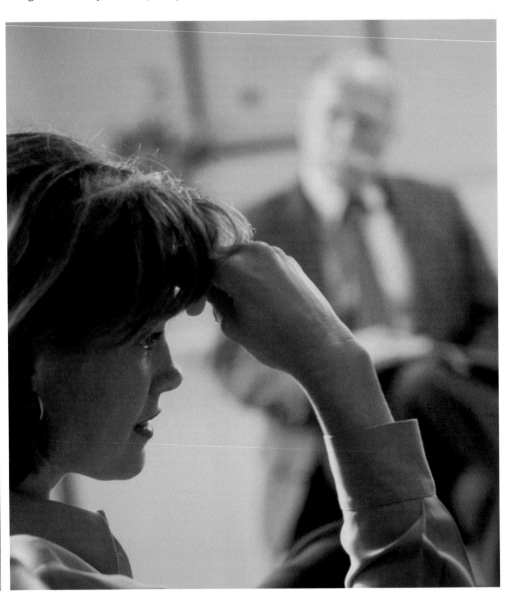

▲ *Pyschotherapy can help to unbury thoughts or feelings that are destructive or are felt to be unacceptable. Once out in the open such feelings can be dealt with.*

unaware of the clock's existence before it stopped. The occasional ability some people seem to possess that enables them to solve a problem in an apparent flash of insight, rather than by conscious thought, also betrays the existence of the subconscious activity of the mind (see Mind).

## Development of a subconscious

From the moment of birth, feelings and images bombard the consciousness, and the mind begins the process of trying to make sense of them and to record them. Some of the images and feelings are almost certainly wrongly recorded and fail to fit later sensations and impressions; additionally, there is far too much information filtering into the brain for items to be recorded individually. Instead, general impressions and rules of behavior begin to be learned. These rules, however, are an individual's rules rather than the rules that someone teaches him or her.

## Subconscious feelings

Later, however, when the experiences and rules of the individual come into conflict with what he or she decides are the wiser and stronger rules of others, his or her rules

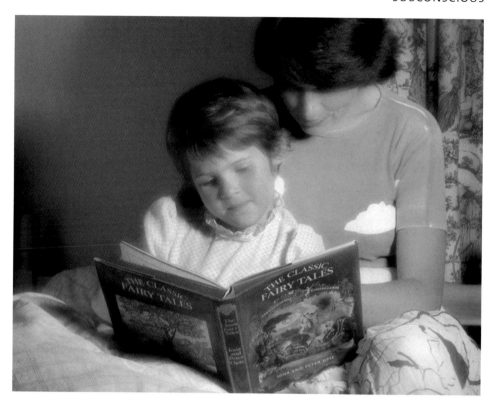

▲ *Fairy tales and folk stories are a possible expression of the most mysterious part of our common experience. They can also act as a focus for nameless childhood fears, and by making them fanciful, diminish them.*

and particular experiences are filed away at the subconscious level. Yet forgetfulness does not prevent a later event from triggering the original feeling or the original reaction, and most people have by chance experienced a sound or a scent that vividly brings back a childhood feeling without being able to place the original event linked to the stimulus.

## Problem solving

Ideas that occur are sorted by the subconscious into sections of the brain and filed as important or unimportant. When the important ideas are brought to conclusions, the subconscious breaks through to the conscious mind with the revelatory facts. This explains why when someone has been seeking the solution to an elusive problem, it can suddenly come unbidden into the mind.

## Racial subconscious

Some of the experiences buried in the subconscious may be common to many people. This led the Swiss psychiatrist Carl Jung to postulate the existence of a racial subconscious that contained a set of memories common to those of a particular ethnic culture. Such a group memory would help to explain how myths, legends, and fairy tales that come from many countries often contain the same elements, even when the people of one country have no direct contact with the inhabitants of another (see Memory).

## Dealing with the subconscious

Most subconscious memories and feelings are harmless enough. However, strong feelings of anger, fear, or desire, which have become buried in a person's subconscious mind because they are regarded as

unacceptable, will almost certainly emerge unexpectedly from time to time as behavior that is destructive to the possessor, or to another person. In such circumstances it must be helpful to draw out from the subconscious the memories and feelings that cause the unfortunate behavior in order that the person may recognize them for what they are and come to terms with them (see Psychotherapy).

This process of examining the subconscious is the basis for many types of psychotherapy, and psychoanalytic therapy in particular. Because present thoughts can sometimes trigger subconscious memories under relaxed conditions, the examination of dreams (for which we seldom feel responsible) and the use of free association are practices that can be of value (see Dreaming). In free association the patient is asked to say whatever comes into his or her head, wandering from image to image with the expectation that any pressure coming from the subconscious will emerge into consciousness by suddenly remembered associations.

## The subconscious and psychotherapy

It must not be assumed, though, that the subconscious mind is the repository of the worst aspects of personality, or thoughts that ought to remain hidden. The subconscious mind is also likely to contain the unexpressed visions of the creative person, and joys and happiness of which we remember little.

Many people who have explored the subconscious through psychotherapy say that the journey can be life-transforming.

See also: Psychiatry; Psychology; Rapid eye movement sleep; Sleep and sleep problems

# Sudden infant death syndrome

**A friend lost her baby and was told it was a case of sudden infant death syndrome (SIDS). How can I protect my baby?**

All you can do is care for your baby as well as possible, and follow basic safety measures. You can learn about baby care at prenatal classes. Try to breast-feed, because this can help the baby's overall health. The baby should sleep in a room that is warm and free from drafts, and should never be allowed to get too hot or cold. You can check a baby's body temperature by feeling under the crib covers. If the baby is sweaty, he or she is too hot and will need a drink of cool water. If you or your partner smoke, try to quit, and never smoke in a room where your baby is, because smoking is thought to have a link with SIDS. SIDS is rare, but always consult your doctor if your baby seems unwell.

**My sister lost her baby of four weeks through SIDS. She is now pregnant again. What is the risk that SIDS will happen twice?**

The chance that this tragic event will occur again is very slight, although, understandably, many parents have a great fear of losing another baby in the same way. The chance of a second SIDS in the same family is no greater than the chance of a first SIDS in another family.

**Is it true that I should not put my baby on her stomach to sleep, because of the possibility of suffocation?**

No one knows what causes SIDS. Doctors advise that babies sleep on their back. Do not put your baby to sleep facedown. There should be no pillows in the crib.

**Despite continuing research, the cause of SIDS is still unexplained. However, parents can take several measures to reduce the risk to their baby. Position and temperature are important factors.**

There is nothing more tragic and disturbing for a family than the unexpected and unexplained death of a baby. An apparently healthy baby is put to bed in a crib or carriage. When next looked at, he or she is dead, and for no obvious reason.

This sad phenomenon, known as SIDS (sudden infant death syndrome), is one of the most pressing and perplexing problems facing doctors. Some of the contributing factors that are thought to cause the syndrome are poor prenatal care, low birth weight, and exposure of the fetus to alcohol and tobacco. There are about 2,500 deaths from SIDS per year in the United States, but there has been a 52 percent reduction of SIDS deaths from 1990 to 2000. Educational programs produced by the American SIDS Institute have effected this reduction in deaths, and it is hoped that additional research will eliminate deaths or at least reduce them further.

Sudden infant death syndrome is most common among babies aged between four weeks and one year, and they occur particularly between the ages of two and four months. There are more cases among boys, twins, and babies whose birth weight was low. SIDS also happens more during the autumn and winter (often coinciding with local epidemics of flu), and happens more often to babies who are bottle-fed rather than breast-fed.

There are no warning signs, and death can occur in the parent's bedroom, in hospitals, in clinics—even while a baby is being nursed in its mother's arms.

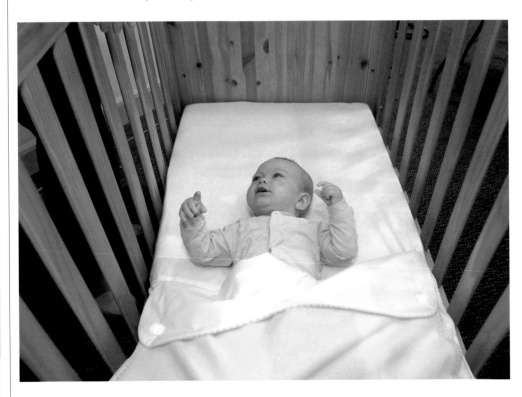

▲ *The recommended position for a young baby is on his or her back with the feet at the foot of the crib, so that the baby cannot wriggle downward under the bedcovers. The number of bedcovers should be appropriate for the temperature of the room.*

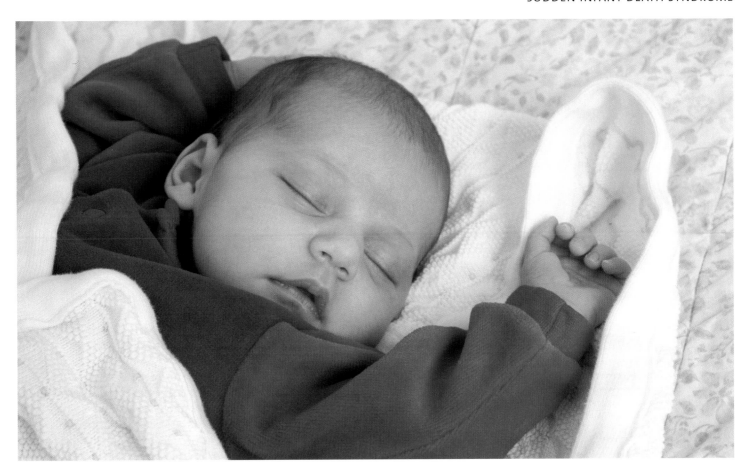

## Symptoms

Probably one of the most puzzling aspects is that there appear to be no warning signals of any kind, but subsequent examination does reveal evidence of unsuspected abnormality or serious disease, such as pneumonia or meningitis, in about one-third of cases. However, recent research has shown that while some babies definitely do die quite inexplicably, the majority have had minor symptoms in the preceding week or 24 hours. These may include a cold, a stuffed-up nose, listlessness, drowsiness, or difficulties with breathing. These minor symptoms are the basis of the apnea, or cessation of breathing, theory. Periods of apnea alternate with active breathing as a normal occurrence during sleep. Some adults, and even more babies, naturally experience this. Usually a baby automatically changes to active breathing by taking a deep breath, but it is possible that some babies who have experienced these minor symptoms do not switch over to active breathing—with fatal results. Crib deaths are not related to choking, smothering, child abuse, or neglect. Contrary to popular belief, many of these babies have been better cared for than those who survive.

## Sleeping positions

Although babies appear to sleep more deeply and wake less if they sleep on their stomach, The American SIDS Institute states that in this position, infants retain more heat than they do when sleeping on their back. Also, babies who sleep facedown are more likely to have apnea (pauses in breathing), and their blood levels of carbon dioxide can rise because they rebreathe the air that they have just exhaled. The American SIDS Institute claims that sleeping on the stomach has up to 12.9 times the risk of death as sleeping on the back.

▲ *For safety, young babies should always be placed in the crib lying on their back.*

## Immunization and SIDS

On March 12, 2003, the Institute of Medicine (IOM) published a report called *Immunization Safety Review: Vaccinations and Sudden Unexpected Death in Infancy.* The report sought to discover if the use of vaccines contributed to an increased risk of SIDS. The report concluded that there was no reason to believe that vaccines given to infants during their first year of life contribute to an increased risk of SIDS, and that in fact routine vaccinations protected infants from many potentially dangerous diseases.

## Research into SIDS

Although SIDS has declined by about 40 percent since it was advised that babies sleep on their back, research is ongoing to discover any major abnormalities associated with SIDS, to identify possible tests that will prevent the syndrome, and to find which factors during pregancy put infants at greater risk of SIDS.

## Effects on the family

For the parents, profound shock is probably the first reaction, then feelings of guilt. Older children, who may have felt jealous of the baby, also suffer from guilt. The entire family should talk to an understanding outsider. Comfort and practical help during this time of grief can be sought from friends, the family doctor, a health visitor, a therapist, or a religious counselor.

*See also:* **Prenatal care**

# Suffocation

**Suffocation is a medical emergency in which the body's airways are prevented from conducting oxygen to the lungs, through accident, a blockage of the airway by a foreign body, or disease.**

## Questions and Answers

**Can someone suffocate by swallowing his or her tongue?**

Yes. If someone swallows the tongue and blocks the internal airways, suffocation will result unless first aid measures are given immediately. You should not try to pull the tongue back into its correct position. Lie the person on his or her back with the head tilted backward. Pull the chin forward so that the tongue falls backward and creates a space through which air can flow, then give mouth-to-mouth resuscitation if necessary, and keep the chin forward at all costs until expert help arrives. Never leave the victim unattended.

**My daughter sleeps with her head under the blankets. Am I right to worry that she might suffocate?**

It is very unlikely that your daughter will be at any risk from suffocation by sleeping in this way. Not only are blankets porous, but if the waste carbon dioxide built up to a dangerous level in your daughter's blood, her body's natural defense mechanism would come into operation and force her to come up for air in good time.

**I was in a very crowded train and worried that I might be suffocated. Would this have been possible, and could I have prevented it?**

Being pressed in a crowd can be frightening and dangerous too. If you feel there is a real risk of suffocation, position your hands near your face to create an air space between you and the next person. Or try to make movements with your head to create the same effect. Above all, don't panic, since this could endanger your own safety and that of other people in the crowd. Panic can quickly infect a crowd.

Suffocation has a variety of causes, but common to all is that the body is deprived of oxygen. Normally, as a breath is taken in through the mouth or nose, air enters the body and travels down a series of tubes to expand the lungs. To help make lung expansion possible, the ribs are pulled up and out and the muscular diaphragm below the lungs is pulled downward. In tiny sacs (alveoli) in the lungs, the oxygen in air breathed in is exchanged for waste carbon dioxide. Oxygen now enters the bloodstream and, assisted by the pumping of the heart, is carried to all parts of the body. Gas rich in carbon dioxide is breathed out as the rib cage contracts and the diaphragm retracts upward (see Breathing; Diaphragm).

About 16 times a minute, for an entire lifetime, this mechanism continues without the need for conscious control. The body also has a built-in emergency mechanism designed to protect vital organs from lack of oxygen, particularly the brain, in which cells begin to die after only five minutes without oxygen. If for some reason the amount of oxygen in the blood falls and the carbon dioxide content rises, this change is monitored by cells in the brain. In response, breathing becomes deeper and more rapid, and the blood vessels to all but essential areas are shut down. If necessary and possible, the body moves to a situation where more oxygen is available.

Despite the body's fail-safe mechanism, suffocation can occur from within the body if the airway is so obstructed that oxygen is prevented from reaching the alveoli or, having reached them, is prevented from reaching the blood. Choking on swallowed objects, swallowing the tongue in accidents, swelling of the tissues of the airways as a result of disease, or an intense allergic reaction can all cause suffocation. Even if oxygen enters the lungs, suffocation will result

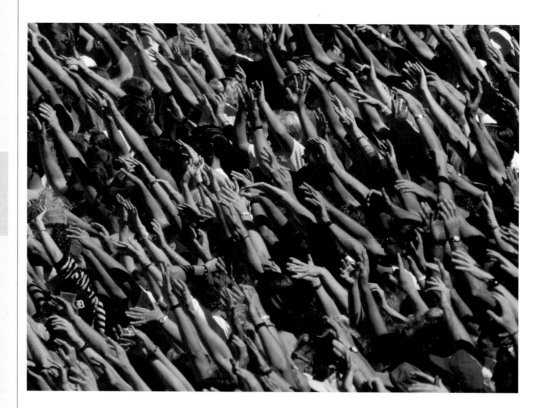

▲ *In crowded places such as bleachers in sports venues, there is a danger of suffocation if someone trips and gets trapped underneath other people.*

if the lung tissues are damaged and cannot exchange oxygen for carbon dioxide.

All diseases of the lungs and airways can cause suffocation. These include asthma and bronchitis, which narrow the airways; emphysema, which overdistends and may partially destroy the alveoli; and cancer, which eats its way into normal lung tissue. In patients suffering from pneumonia, oxygen is sometimes prevented from entering the bloodstream (see Lung and Lung Diseases).

Suffocation from forces operating outside the body is usually the result of some kind of accident. The nose and mouth, the exit and entry points of the airway, may be blocked if someone is crushed in an accident. A strangling constriction of some kind around the neck can also cause suffocation.

## Symptoms

The exact symptoms of suffocation depend on its cause, but there are standard signs to look for. If there is some kind of obstruction, the neck muscles may make enormous, powerful contractions in an attempt to get rid of the blockage. At the same time, breathing will be labored and noisy and a bubbly fluid, possibly pink or red in color, may emerge from between the patient's lips. Other signs are a gradual increase in blueness of the skin, progressively deeper and more rapid breathing, and, after a time, a lapse into unconsciousness. When this happens, breathing may stop; at this point first aid is vital to prevent death or brain damage. The brain cannot live long without a continuous supply of oxygenated blood

## First aid measures

If a victim's airway is blocked from the outside, or the chest is being crushed, an attempt must be made to remove the obstruction or free the victim from a trapped position.

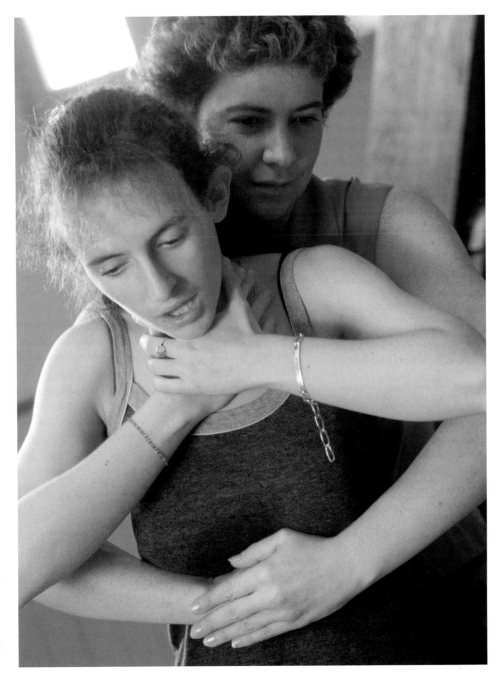

▲ *When someone is suffocating because of an obstruction, abdominal thrusts, known as the Heimlich maneuver, can be performed to dislodge the obstruction.*

## Heimlich maneuver

If there is an obstruction inside the body, and the patient is still conscious, the Heimlich maneuver should be attempted. The rescuer stands behind the victim and places both arms just above his or her belt line. The victim's head, arms, and upper torso should hang forward. The rescuer should press a fist firmly inward and upward into the victim's abdomen, to try to dislodge the obstruction. Or, the victim should be asked to cough as hard as possible to try to dislodge the obstruction, and to breathe as slowly and deeply as possible. If this fails, the rescuer could try to scoop out the obstruction using two fingers.

If the patient is weak or unconscious, artificial respiration should be started by the mouth-to-mouth method. Speed is essential; a life

is at risk and after five minutes there is a risk of brain damage caused by a lack of oxygen.

A rescuer must call for help without stopping artificial respiration or leaving the patient unattended. If alone, a rescuer should shout out as loudly as possible between breaths into the patient's lungs—or try to pull the victim toward a door, a window, or a telephone so that medical help can be summoned without placing the victim at any further risk. Sometimes, an obstruction gets into the lungs and even though the person may be breathing freely, there may be wheezing or a cough. In this case, medical help should be sought immediately.

> *See also:* Allergies; Oxygen; Unconsciousness

# Sugars

**Do glucose tablets and drinks provide instant energy?**

No. Glucose is the fuel that gives the body energy, but it does not instantly provide energy. Glucose is absorbed into the body and stored in the liver and muscles as glycogen until it is required. The amount of glucose found in the blood is small (0.1 percent of the blood is glucose), and more is added from the glycogen store when blood sugar levels drop. All carbohydrates convert to glucose, so there is no need to take glucose tablets and drinks.

**Why do diabetics have to restrict their sugar intake?**

A diabetic diet consists of a controlled amount of all carbohydrates. Diabetes is caused by the inability of the body to control the amount of sugar in the blood, so the diet aims to provide the patient with the exact amount of carbohydrates needed.

**My children eat lots of candy. Will it affect their teeth?**

Yes. Sugary and starchy foods provide a breeding ground for bacteria; they tend to produce acid substances that attack the protective enamel of the teeth. Once the enamel barrier is breached, the problem becomes worse. Encourage your children not to eat so much candy, and make sure they brush their teeth to get rid of the bacteria.

**Is brown sugar better for you than ordinary white sugar?**

Brown sugar is virtually the same as white sugar, but it has not had all the impurities removed. White sugar is produced by chemical processing. The basic constituent of sugar is sucrose. Brown sugar is almost pure sucrose.

**Sugar has other uses as well as sweetening foods and drinks. In various forms, sugar plays a vital role in providing energy for the body—and the body's preferred source of energy is the sugar glucose.**

The major part of a balanced diet consists of carbohydrates, which are sugars and starches. Carbohydrates contain atoms of carbon, hydrogen, and oxygen in varying configurations and it is the arrangements of these atoms that give the different carbohydrates their specific properties and names. Single sugar units or simple sugars are called monosaccharides, such as glucose. Disaccharides such as sucrose, lactose, and maltose are formed from two single saccharide molecules bonded together; they are the sugars normally found in foods. Polysaccharides, such as starches and glycogen, are long chains of glucose molecules.

## Sugar and digestion

During digestion, carbohydrates are broken down into simple sugars, especially glucose, which can be absorbed into the body and used as fuel to provide energy for all metabolic processes (see Digestive System). The glucose absorbed into the body is not all poured into the bloodstream after being digested; a certain amount is diverted to the liver where it is converted into glycogen, or animal starch (see Starch). The liver acts as an energy store for the body (see Liver and Liver Diseases). When instant energy is required, the liver converts some of the stored glycogen into glucose and releases it into the bloodstream. Thus, a high-glucose meal has no special energy-giving properties, because the excess is simply stored. Even if there is a temporary lack of carbohydrate, the liver is able to synthesize glucose from fats and proteins (see Glucose).

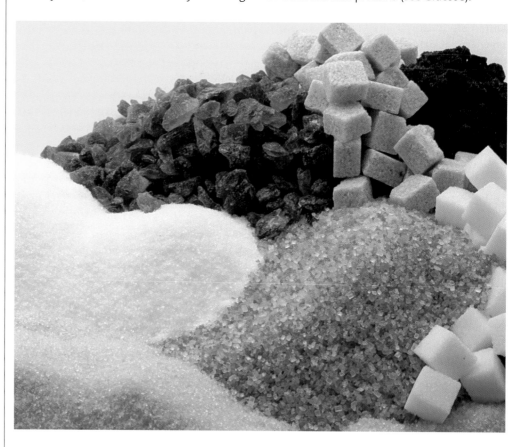

▲ *White sugar is pure sucrose and brown sugars are virtually the same. It is their impurities that give brown sugars their color.*

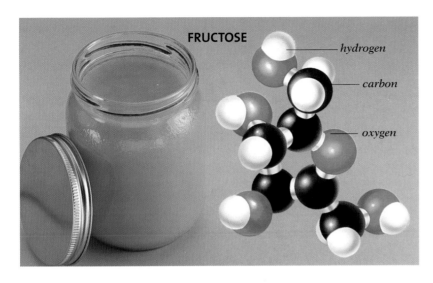

▲ *The simple sugars (monosaccharides) are commonly found in natural foods. Fructose, found in honey, is a prime example.*

uneasiness, and sweating; it may even lead to epileptic fits or unconsciousness. Usually, people who suffer from hypoglycemia learn to recognize the symptoms and eat a sugar-rich food to arrest the problem (see Hypoglycemia).

## Sugars and health

Although a certain amount of sugar is useful in that it contributes to providing energy for the body, an excess of sugar can also lead to harmful effects. These include obesity and tooth decay (see Obesity; Teeth and Teething). In addition, sugar is thought by some to be a contributory factor in hardening of the arteries (see Arteries and Artery Disease).

There is a certain amount of evidence that an excess of sugar in the diet, along with smoking and a high fat intake, can contribute to atherosclerosis (see Fats; Smoking). Also, sugar is a very potent source of calories, and people with a tendency to obesity should avoid pure sugar. Although all the starchy food that is eaten is converted to simple sugar in the body, for a steady supply of energy it is best to eat

## Blood sugar

The blood contains about 0.1 percent glucose, and this continuously supplies the energy needs of the body tissues. It is particularly important to the brain, which has no means of storing fuel. For this reason, it is crucial that the concentration of sugar in the blood is monitored and regulated. Several hormones, of which insulin is the most important, are involved in the fine control necessary to attain the correct balance between the instant availability and storage of glucose (see Insulin). When the level of sugar in the blood rises, the pancreas releases insulin to the bloodstream and this enables glucose to be stored or used by the tissues. Too little insulin, or a total lack of it, leads to high concentrations of blood sugar; this condition is called diabetes mellitus, or sugar diabetes (see Diabetes).

On the other hand, an overproduction of insulin leads to a condition called hypoglycemia, which results from too little sugar in the blood. This condition quickly impairs brain function, leading to such symptoms as hunger,

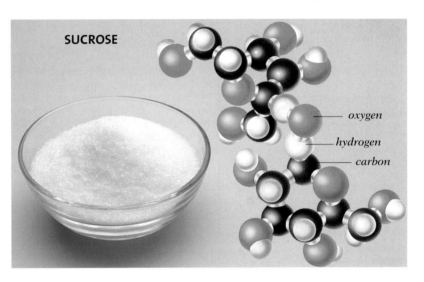

▲ *When two simple sugar molecules join together a disaccharide is formed. Ordinary table sugar (sucrose) is the best-known.*

complex carbohydrates, such as brown rice, grains, and other whole foods. Digestion of these foods takes longer and the slow absorption of sugars provides a constant supply of energy and limits the amount of sugar converted into fat and thereby stored. This helps to guard against atherosclerosis. In general, a healthy diet should contain more starch, less fat, and little refined sugar.

Sugary foods are thought to cause dental caries. In fact, sugars can have an effect on dental health, but indirectly. The mouth is a breeding ground for bacteria, which will feed off sugars or starches left clinging to the teeth and produce acid waste products that attack and etch the teeth, producing cavities.

Finally, carbohydrates do not require oxygen to convert them to energy, so they fuel exercises involving muscular contractions.

**See also: Bacteria; Diet**

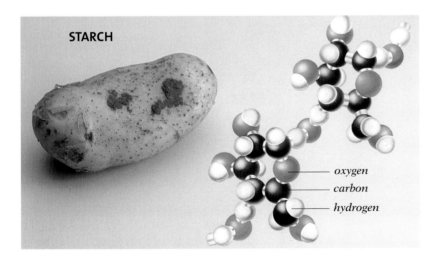

▲ *When many sugar molecules join up, polysaccharides are formed. These are the starches found in vegetables.*

# Suicide

## Questions and Answers

**My sister is frequently depressed and often threatens suicide, but so far she has never attempted it. Should I take her threats seriously?**

It is a common error to think that those who talk about suicide never do it. Her suicidal threats are an expression of her obvious distress, and treatment for her depression should be sought before she does something drastic. Ask your doctor to recommend professional help.

**Is it true that the suicide rate is higher among artists and writers?**

There is a high rate of suicide in all jobs that place a lot of pressure on the achievement of the individual. However, the majority of suicides occur among older people, the less well off, the unemployed, and the physically ill.

**My friend's son committed suicide, and later it was learned that he was bullied in school. Could his suicide have been prevented?**

Possibly. Many suicides would not take place if the distressed person had been able to talk about his or her problems. However, many factors usually contribute to drive an individual to suicide, and although the bullying may have been an important one, it may not have been the only one.

**Why do many women make repeated suicide attempts?**

It is thought that more women survive an attempted suicide because of their tendency to use less violent methods than men (poisoning, for example), leaving a chance of survival. It has also been suggested that women use the appeal effect of a suicide attempt more because other methods of exerting pressure or displaying aggression are not in their nature.

**Most people have moments of despair and self-hatred, but only a small number of them will actually attempt or commit suicide. What drives people to it, and what help is available for people who have reached the breaking point?**

Many factors can contribute to causing the depression, despair, or low self-esteem that drive a person to suicide. Suicidal individuals are now recognized as either being ill or in great distress, and should receive help and treatment before it is too late.

### Who commits suicide?

More men commit suicide than women, but a far greater number of women make unsuccessful attempts to kill themselves. Studies show that virtually no children below the age of 15 commit suicide, but the rate tends to increase steadily as people get older (see Aging). Divorced and widowed people are far more likely to kill themselves than married or single people. People with strong family, community, or religious ties are less prone to suicide.

Suicide is more frequent among the professional classes (managers, executives, doctors, and businessmen) and among low-status unskilled workers than among the skilled workers who form the middle group of the population. People living in small country towns are among the least likely to kill themselves. Those living in big cities, especially in the city center rather than in the suburbs, are most at risk.

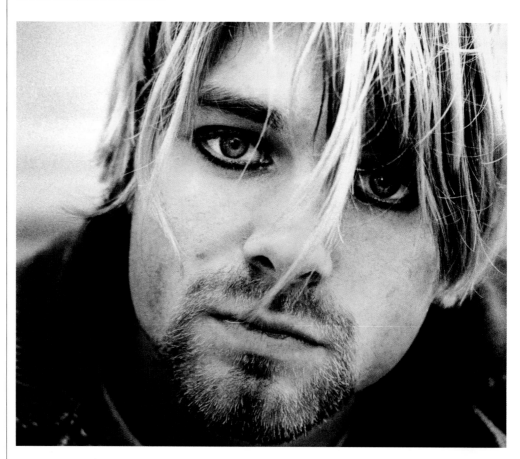

▲ *Nirvana frontman Kurt Cobain committed suicide in 1994. As with many suicides, there was a clear warning of the approaching tragedy. Six weeks before he fatally shot himself in his Seattle home, Cobain went into a coma after overdosing on a cocktail of painkillers and champagne while in Rome, Italy, on tour.*

More people commit suicide in spring and early summer than at any other time of the year, and there are often more deaths during public holidays, when the lonely feel even lonelier. The low rate of suicide in wartime has been explained by the closer involvement of the individual with the group, family, or community during that time.

## Why?

Contrary to popular belief, suicide is not generally the result of a rational weighing of the pros and cons of living. Though an individual may have had suicidal thoughts, the final decision to kill him- or herself is usually made impulsively under severe emotional stress (see Stress).

Usually there is a combination of factors that drives an otherwise stable person over the edge into the desperate act of suicide. A major misfortune or life change, such as the end of a marriage or relationship, the death of a loved one, or the loss of a job, may trigger the despair that precedes suicide. Social factors have been found to contribute to suicide in two-thirds of cases; in one-third of suicides they were the principal cause.

Nearly a third of those who kill themselves are physically ill. It has been estimated that for one in five of all suicide cases poor physical

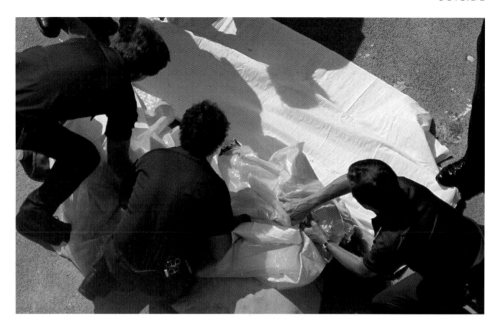

▲ *For every person who commits suicide there are 25 who attempt suicide but survive, because the method chosen is not effective or they are rescued in time.*

health was the primary reason for the action. An unhappy love affair appears to be the motivation for suicide in only one out of 20 cases, and failed examinations or pregnancy out of wedlock are even less common as a cause.

Loneliness and alienation from the community are an important cause of suicide. The person who kills him- or herself is likely to experience a high degree of isolation and separation from the society he or she lives in. High rates of suicide are found where communities have disintegrated and are unstable, and where the needs of the individual are not satisfied.

The majority of those who kill themselves are severely depressed, and indeed a similar psychological state underlies depression and suicide. In both cases, the individual turns against him- or herself hostile impulses that were originally meant for other people. If he or she is unable to express angry or aggressive feelings externally, they may turn into self-aggression, which is expressed as self-criticism and self-hatred, or in the more extreme actions of self-injury and self-destruction in the case of a potential suicide.

Alongside the urge toward self-destruction, there is frequently a contrasting urge toward human contact and communication with other people. Suicides know their act will affect others, and usually they give warning before or during a suicide attempt. Sometimes an individual may use the act of suicide as a means of forcing others to express their love and concern for him or her.

The aged, the poor, and the physically sick make up a large proportion of those who kill themselves, and who are particularly vulnerable. Those living away from their family group are also more likely to commit suicide than others. The rate of suicide increases with age and the peak age for suicide is over 84 years.

Marriage and a big family have been linked with a lower rate of suicide but a higher rate of homicide, often a family crime. The impersonal life of the big city has been blamed for the large number of suicides, especially among immigrants and those living alone. Poor areas with a highly mobile population show the highest rates of all worldwide.

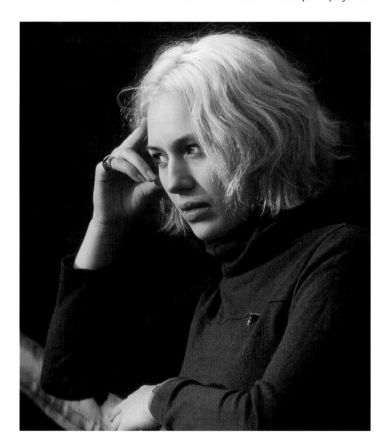

▲ *Suicide is very often preceded by depression. Young women are the most likely to attempt a suicide that is unsuccessful.*

## Questions and Answers

**Someone I knew committed suicide last month after he lost his job. Is there really any link between unemployment and suicide?**

The change of life that occurs when a person loses a job, and the consequent loss of self-esteem, disorientation, and isolation from the community, may trigger a depression that leads to suicide. However, it is not possible to generalize from this and say that there is a close relationship between economic climate and levels of suicide. Many other factors will always come into play.

**Why do some people make suicide pacts?**

Most people who make suicide pacts are not young unhappy lovers but older married couples, particularly when one may have a serious illness. Pacts, which are extremely rare, are illegal, and a survivor may be charged with the criminal offense of aiding and abetting the suicide of the other.

**A friend recently took an overdose of pills, but it was not fatal. Will she do it again?**

Those who have attempted suicide are more at risk of suicide than any other members of the population, especially during the first four years after the attempt. The likelihood of a second attempt depends on whether the situation that caused the first attempt has improved.

**Does a person's religion or cultural background play any part in determining whether he or she might commit suicide?**

In some cultures suicide has been admired: for example, some Eastern religions have honored people choosing to free themselves from their bodies. In contrast, the Jewish and Christian religions condemned suicide as sinful. However, modern attitudes in many countries have moved toward seeing suicide as a psychological and social problem.

## Suicide statistics for the United States (2001)

A total number of 30,622 people committed suicide in one year, meaning that an average of 83.9 people committed suicide per day—about 1 person every 17.2 minutes.

Suicide was the 11th leading cause of death among adults and it was the third leading cause of death among people aged 15 to 24 years (after accidents and homicide).

Suicides outnumbered homicides by 3 to 2 (there were 20,308 homicides).

A total of 765,000 people attempted suicide.

Males committed suicide at a rate over four times that of females, yet women were three times more likely to attempt suicide than men. Suicide was the eighth leading cause of death among males and the 19th leading cause of death among females.

The elderly (age 65 and over) had rates of suicide of more than 50 percent higher than that of the nation as a whole, with approximately 15 elderly people committing suicide per day—an average of one every 1 hour and 37.5 minutes.

Suicide accounted for 14 percent of deaths among people aged 15 to 24 years, with almost 11 young people committing suicide per day—an average of one every 2 hours and 3.7 minutes. Most suicides by young people take place in their own homes between 3:00 P.M. and midnight.

Firearms were the most common method used for completing suicide, accounting for over 55 percent, followed by hanging or suffocation (20.2 percent), poisoning (17 percent), falls (2.1 percent), cuts (1.5 percent), drowning (1.1 percent), and fire (0.5 percent).

The suicide rate is much higher among the unemployed than among the employed. Heavy drinkers are also particularly vulnerable to attempts at suicide (see Alcoholism). Among people suffering depression, those individuals most at risk are likely to be those undergoing prolonged bouts of insomnia, those who come from a broken home, and those who have already made a previous suicide attempt. They are probably not receiving any psychiatric help (see Psychiatry).

## Methods

Few suicides or attempted suicides are carefully planned. The method used depends on what is available to the individual. In the United States, where guns are relatively easy to obtain, shooting is the most common means of suicide—68 percent of gun-related deaths are suicides. In Great Britain, by contrast, where many kinds of gun are illegal, poisoning accounts for most deaths. Other common methods are hanging and drowning.

Those who survive a suicide attempt may suffer some lasting aftereffects, depending on the method used. Aspirin and acetaminophen can sometimes cause permanent damage to the kidney and liver (see Aspirin and Analgesics; Kidneys and Kidney Diseases; Liver and Liver Diseases). Some drugs taken in large quantities cause permanent brain damage (see Brain Damage and Disease). Survivors of more violent attempts may be left with a physical disability, or may spend some painful days or weeks in a hospital before dying from an indirectly caused ailment such as pneumonia.

## Attempted suicide

For every one person who kills himself, there are at least 25 who attempt suicide and survive. Many more cases are never brought to the hospital, either because the injuries are small or because the individual or his or her family feels ashamed.

While the majority of actual suicides are older men, 65 percent of suicide attempts are made by women, and the rates are highest between 25 and 40 years of age. One-quarter of women

the patient's problems or giving the routine care and support that are vital if the patient is to feel secure, loved, and valued.

A suicide attempt sometimes reveals problems that can then be remedied. The impact that it creates may lead to an improvement in family relations or to the individual's being removed from a socially isolated situation (see Family Relationships). In many cases, it highlights an emotional or physical illness that can be treated. Sometimes the social services of the community can give practical help and advice (see Health Care System).

## Prevention of suicide

In recent years much valuable work in suicide prevention has been done by organizations such as the Samaritans and Lifeline. People in distress can call them at any time and speak in complete confidence to a sympathetic layperson. If appropriate, they may be referred to a doctor. In cities where these organizations operate, surveys have shown a reduction in the suicide rates.

## Living wills and assisted suicides

For many people the right to die is an important part of human dignity. Some people who are terminally ill, for example, believe they have a right to end their own life if the quality of life sinks below what they consider bearable. Others argue, often from

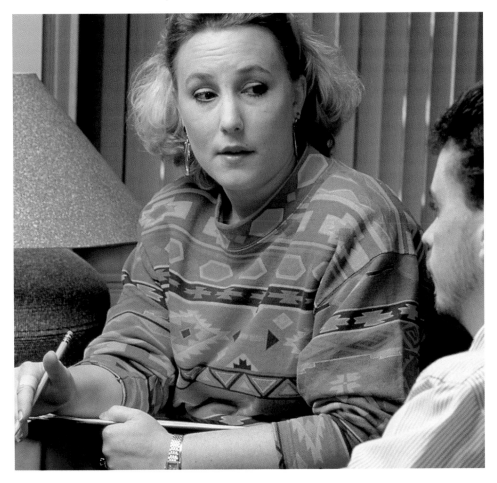

▲ *For many people who survive a suicide attempt, sympathetic counseling may be all they need to help them come to terms with their problems.*

who try to kill themselves are between the ages of 15 and 24; many of them take an overdose of pills because they feel unable to cope or because they experience a sense of failure after separating from a boyfriend or husband.

In the past, those who attempted suicide were often branded as attention seekers who were making a gesture to manipulate others without any genuine intention of killing themselves. However, recent research has shown that apparently harmless acts of self-injury are often followed by more dangerous acts, and that 15 percent of those who attempt suicide afterward succeed in killing themselves. More than 10 percent of those who commit suicide had previously made several attempts. It is now recognized that the cry for help of the attempted suicide generally represents a sincere statement of distress.

## Treatment

Although many doctors will prescribe antidepressant drugs to tide an individual over a period of crisis, the only long-term cure is for the patient to receive some kind of psychotherapy. He or she will then be able to discuss any problems and come to terms with painful or aggressive feelings whose suppression may be responsible for the self-injury (see Psychotherapy).

The doctor or therapist may enlist the cooperation of sympathetic relatives or friends, who can very often contribute a great deal to the success of recovery, either providing insights into

a religious viewpoint, that every life is sacred and that no one has the right to take it away. Doctors can sometimes find themselves caught between, on the one hand, their professional duty to preserve a patient's life and, on the other, their respect for a patient's right of self-determination and compassion for his or her suffering.

It is against this background that the phenomenon of the living will has developed. The living will is a document by which individuals let it be known what they would like to happen to them should they no longer be in a position to determine their future—for example, if they were to be permanently brain-damaged or in a coma. Those who have living wills elect not to be kept alive by artificial means if the chances of recovery seem very slight. Living wills have proved ethical and legal minefields, and in some states they are illegal. Before anyone makes a living will, it is important to check with the district attorney's office to find out what position his or her state takes on this issue.

The related issue of assisted suicide (providing help to end the life of somebody who cannot end it himself or herself) is even more contentious. While under strictly defined circumstances it is legal in the Netherlands, it remains illegal throughout the United States. Any person who assists another to commit suicide can be indicted on a charge of homicide.

> *See also:* **Depression; Euthanasia; Overdoses; Poisoning**

# Sunburn

## Questions and Answers

**I am fair-skinned and my friend is dark. Why can she spend a long time in the sun without burning while I have to be very careful?**

Being fair-skinned means that you have little pigment in your skin. Your friend has more pigment, and can also manufacture more than you when exposed to sunlight. She has a natural barrier to the sun's harmful rays, and is capable of developing even greater protection. You will burn easily because your skin cannot produce enough protective pigment and no amount of sunbathing will alter this.

**Can some drugs make you more sensitive to the sun?**

Yes. Examples are the tranquilizer chlorpromazine and the antibiotic oxytetracycline. This abnormal reaction is called photosensitivity. A rash like sunburn develops on areas exposed to the sun, but if the drug is stopped, the rash fades.

**I have very sensitive skin. Is there any treatment I can have before going on vacation this year?**

You could have a course of ultraviolet ray therapy beforehand, to increase your pigmentation. Or you could use a sunscreen preparation that filters out the sun's stronger rays, allowing a slow tan to develop.

**I have fair hair that becomes lighter in the sun while my skin becomes darker. Why is this?**

The pigment in hair is already present, while that in skin appears only when the pigment-producing cells are activated by sunlight. Fair hair has a different sort of pigment from dark hair and, unlike dark hair, light hair becomes bleached on exposure to strong sunlight.

**Deliberately exposing the skin to the sun can be a risky activity. To limit skin damage, common sense and forethought will help prevent not only the discomfort of sunburn but also the danger of developing serious conditions such as skin cancer.**

The sun has traditionally played a beneficent role in human civilization and has been seen in many cultures as a life giver. Attitudes are beginning to change, however. The discovery in the mid-1980s that the ozone layer—the part of the Earth's atmosphere that protects the planet from the sun's harmful ultraviolet radiation—was under assault from synthetic pollutants and that, as a consequence, people increasingly run the risk of developing skin cancer and possibly cataracts from overexposure to the sun's rays, has made people view the sun with more wariness (see Ozone Layer).

### How sunburn occurs

Sunburn is the result of immediate sun damage to the skin. Sunburn is a form of radiation burn rather than heat burn. Unlike a burn caused by heat, sunburn does not completely develop and is not felt until a few hours after it happens.

The sun is really a small star and its energy can be compared with a continuous and enormous atomic explosion. Some of its rays are deadly, but these are filtered out by the Earth's atmosphere and never reach the Earth itself. The rays that do pass through the atmosphere are part of the sun's spectrum, which consists of visible rays that are seen as light; infrared rays that

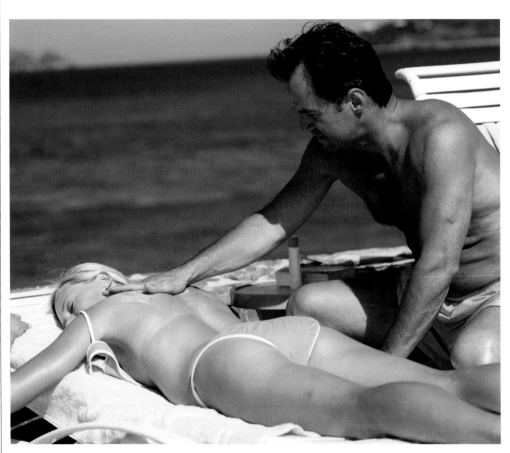

▲ *Although sunbathing on the beach is a relaxing activity, in reality the sun's rays reflecting off water can be extremely damaging to the skin.*

can be felt as heat; and the ultraviolet rays, which cause sunburn. The rays are called ultraviolet because they are positioned beyond the violet end of the visible spectrum.

Both ultraviolet and infrared rays are capable of causing damage to the body. However, infrared rays do not cause a problem, since they are registered as heat, and an exposed area can be withdrawn before any harm is done. It is the ultraviolet rays that cause problems because they can penetrate and damage the skin without giving an immediate feeling of warmth; this results in sunburn.

Ultraviolet rays produce their effect by transferring energy to molecules in the skin, causing a photochemical reaction. The amount of energy released depends on the wavelength of the rays. The shorter wavelengths carry and release more energy than the longer ones, and are more penetrating.

## Effects on the skin

The skin is made up of two layers. In the outer layer (the epidermis), cells are continuously being shed from the surface and replaced by new cells, which are formed in the lowest level of the epidermis. It is in this outer layer that the effects of sunburn occur (see Skin and Skin Diseases).

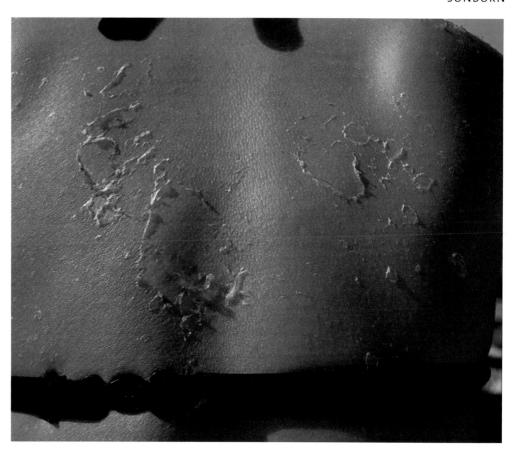

▲ *A tan does not prevent sunburn. Once the pigment-producing skin cells have been saturated with ultraviolet light, further exposure results in radiation burn.*

The bottom (basal) layer of the epidermis contains pigment-producing cells or melanocytes. These are stimulated by ultraviolet light to produce the pigment melanin, which acts as a very efficient filter of the ultraviolet rays (see Melanin). The new pigmentation (which is seen as a suntan) begins soon after exposure to the sun and builds gradually during continual exposure. After a period of exposure, the pigmentation will fade at varying rates, and is likely to disappear within nine months. Sunburn occurs when there is not enough pigment filter present.

## Sunburn cells

There are two types of sun damage: immediate and delayed. The immediate type of damage is sunburn, but, as with other radiation burns, its effects do not show for some hours. The first signs are redness and a sensation of burning caused by an increase in the blood supply to the skin. This may happen anytime up to 24 hours after exposure. Later, small blisters may develop (see Blisters).

More severe damage produces larger blisters and can actually damage some of the cells in the epidermis. These damaged cells are called sunburn cells. The degree of sunburn depends on the strength of the ultraviolet rays.

## Long-term sun damage

Sunburn itself is not as serious as the long-term damage to the skin. This is caused by repeated sun damage to the cells at the skin's surface and to the supporting tissues below. It takes years to develop, but once it has happened it is irreversible (see Wrinkles).

The changes are similar to those of aging (see Aging), and the obvious effects can be seen in a sailor's or land worker's face, where there is marked wrinkling and a leathery thickening of the skin. Other effects can be very localized, such as patchy increases in the pigmentation and a thickening of the horny covering of the skin. This can give rise to wartlike lumps, called solar keratoses, which are common in the middle-aged and elderly. Widening of the blood vessels of the face and dryness and cracking of the skin are part of the aging process but are more marked in people who have spent their lives outdoors exposed to weather and to the sun.

## Skin cancer

The most serious risk that can result from repeated overexposure to the sun is skin cancer (see Cancer). The high incidence in the 21st century of skin cancer among people of northern European descent can be directly related to the fact that for the first time they live in areas of bright sunshine. By contrast, skin cancer was very uncommon in the Victorian era, when there was little exposure of the skin. Today, it occurs frequently in sun-worshiping regions like California or Australia. Australia currently has the highest incidence of skin cancer in the world.

People who have had several episodes of sunburn are much more likely to develop skin cancer than those who have never suffered sunburn. However, skin cancer occurs also in people with long-term sun exposure who have never suffered sunburn.

▶ *In the Victorian era, a pale skin was considered a sign of refinement and, in women, of beauty. This, and concealment of the body, almost certainly explains the low incidence of skin cancer over the general population.*

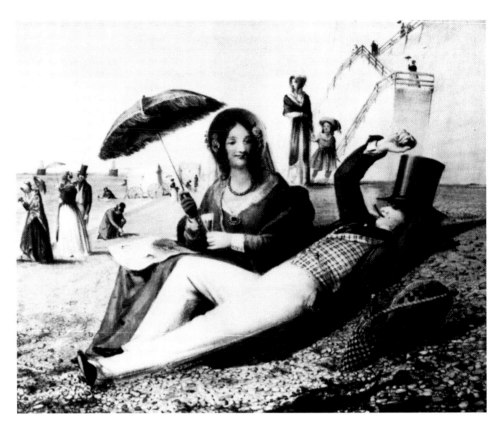

Fair-skinned people who can produce enough melanin pigment to get a good tan are still vulnerable to skin cancer. There is a limit to the number of harmful rays that can be absorbed by the pigment filter, and once this has been saturated these rays can then cause damage. It is therefore not impossible for a tanned person to develop sunburn from excessive exposure. Dark-skinned people can also suffer the same effects but to a much lesser degree.

Children are at particular risk from sunburn. Repeated exposures to sunburn during childhood increase the likelihood of skin cancer during adulthood.

## Treatment

Once sunburn has occurred, the most important factor in treatment is to prevent further damage by avoiding further exposure. In mild burns the redness and burning usually resolve in a few days, and are often followed by peeling. Soothing lotions such as calamine are most effective, and if sleep is disturbed antihistamines may be prescribed. These are mildly sedative but have no effect on the skin.

In more severe burns, the symptoms are usually most acute on the second day when blisters may form on the affected areas. Steroid ointments reduce inflammation as well as the intensity and duration of the skin reaction.

## Prevention

Most people quickly learn how much sun they can take without burning. The body's natural protection is, of course, a tan built up every day by gradually increasing the periods of exposure.

The intensity of the sun must also be taken into account. The most accurate way of gauging this is not by the degree of heat or light, but by the angle of the sun above the horizon. This determines the amount of ultraviolet light that reaches the skin. At midday, the sun is directly overhead and the rays pass through less of the Earth's atmosphere. When the sun is low, in the morning and evening, the strength of the ultraviolet rays is considerably reduced. People are therefore less likely to get sunburned in the early morning or after midafternoon. The danger period is thus roughly 10 A.M. to 3 P.M., when exposure should be kept to a minimum.

Particular care should be taken in swimming, sailing, or skiing. Water absorbs the heat rays but the ultraviolet rays are still being directed onto the skin; and snow gives a feeling of coolness but actually reflects the ultraviolet rays.

There are many sunscreen creams and lotions available that can help to prevent sunburn. Both the American Academy of

| Recommendations of the American Academy of Dermatology and the Skin Cancer Foundation to help reduce the risk of skin cancer and sunburn |
|---|
| Keep exposure to the sun to a minimum at midday and between 10 A.M. and 3 P.M. |
| Apply sunscreen with at least a skin protection factor (SPF) of 15, or higher, to all areas of the body that are exposed to the sun. Reapply the sunscreen every two hours, even on cloudy days, and after swimming or perspiring. |
| Wear clothing that covers the body. Hats should have wide brims to shade both the face and the neck. |
| Avoid exposure to ultraviolet radiation from sunlamps. |
| Children should be protected from excessive exposure to the sun when radiation is strongest (10 A.M. to 3 P.M.). Sunscreen should be applied liberally and frequently to children aged six months or older. Sunscreen should not, however, be used on babies under six months. |
| For babies under six months, keep exposure to sunlight to an absolute minimum, and apply sunscreen. |

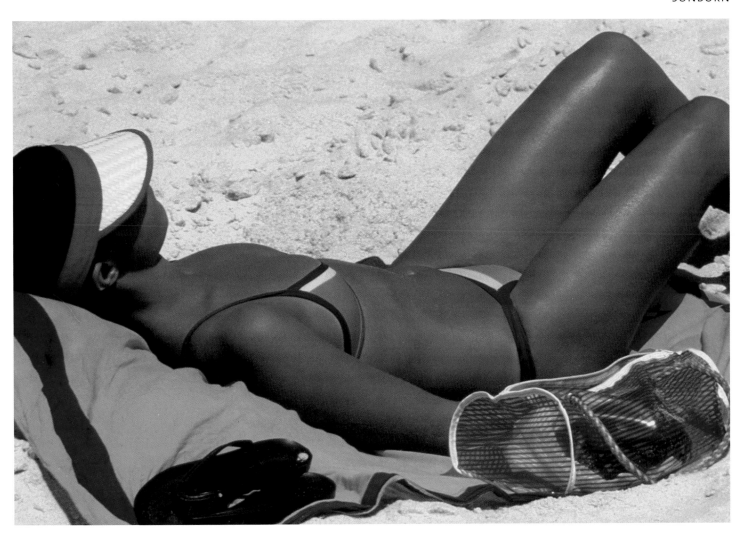

▲ *For much of the 20th century, there was a fashion for gaining a highly prized tan, often at the expense of health. We are now turning full circle: pale skin is becoming acceptable, even fashionable, again.*

Dermatology, and the Skin Cancer Foundation, advise that sunscreen preparations should be applied frequently, and especially just before and after swimming. They protect mainly against the sun's rays but, depending on their strength (sunscreen factor), will let through enough of the longer ultraviolet waves to produce a gradual tan. The tan is, however, no deeper than one obtained simply by gradual exposure without a sunscreen. Some sunscreens give almost total protection by stopping all the ultraviolet and visible rays, so that prolonged exposure without skin damage is possible.

Some parts of the body are more prone to sunburn than others because they are exposed the most. A bald head and the face, nose, tops of the ears, forearms, and backs of the hands are particularly at risk. A hat should always be worn when the hair is thin, and this will also protect the nose and tops of the ears. Otherwise, a sunscreen should be used on these small areas. Clothing is an efficient filter of the sun's harmful rays, if it is opaque.

Children should be protected and must always wear a hat when they are playing out in the sun, and sunblock should be applied liberally and frequently to exposed areas of skin. If possible, children should not be allowed to stay out in the sun for prolonged periods between 10 A.M. and 3 P.M. However, sunscreen should not be used on babies of six months or less, who should rather be kept out of strong sunlight altogether.

## Outlook

In the future people will increasingly have to become more sun-conscious and protect themselves and their children against the possible negative effects of sunburn. However, it is important to remember that not all the effects of ultraviolet light are harmful. Sunlight is essential for health (see Vitamin C; Vitamin D), and perhaps even emotional well-being (see Seasonal Affective Disorder). A healthy glowing skin can make someone feel lively and happy, whereas dull, gloomy weather has a depressant effect.

## Photosensitivity

Some people have excessive sensitivity to the sun which can cause a red, painful rash, scaly skin, and itchy blisters. In severe cases, the person has to avoid going outdoors in daylight. Treatment is with steroids or antihistamines and with desensitization to ultraviolet light, and the sufferer has to wear a high-factor sunblock.

> *See also:* **Dermatology, Eyes and eyesight; Heat and heat disorders; Immune system; Inflammation; Melanoma; Pain; Photosensitivity; Prickly heat; Scars; Steroids**

# Sunstroke

**If you go to a hot country, do you get acclimatized so that you are at less risk of sunstroke?**

Yes, you do. However, it takes several weeks or even months for someone to get acclimatized to the heat. To a large extent, this depends on the amount of physical effort that is required in the heat. It is going to take much longer to be able to carry out strenuous work in the heat than it is if you are just going to take it easy. It is not clear exactly what changes are going on in the body during the period of acclimatization, although there is probably some increase in the efficiency of the sweat glands. Research suggests that a newcomer to the heat loses more salt in sweat than someone who has become used to the heat.

**Is there any difference between sunstroke and heatstroke?**

No. Both terms describe the serious and potentially fatal condition that can occur if the body is excessively heated, resulting in the total breakdown of the temperature-regulating mechanism in the body. Heatstroke, however, is a more accurate name because you can suffer from its effects away from the sun. Heatstroke is a serious problem in some South African mines. If the temperature is high enough, you can get heatstroke even if you're not in direct sun.

**Does prickly heat make you more prone to sunstroke?**

Prickly heat occurs when the skin becomes so hot that the skin cells swell and block the sweat glands, resulting in an itchy rash of tiny, red blisters. Prickly heat is actually very common, and doesn't really indicate any serious trouble. There is one form of heat exhaustion that is often preceded by an episode of prickly heat, but it is nowhere near as severe as heatstroke itself.

**Sunstroke is a dangerous condition that occurs when the body's thermostat breaks down from overheating. Care must be taken in extreme heat, since, even with treatment, sunstroke can be fatal or cause permanent damage.**

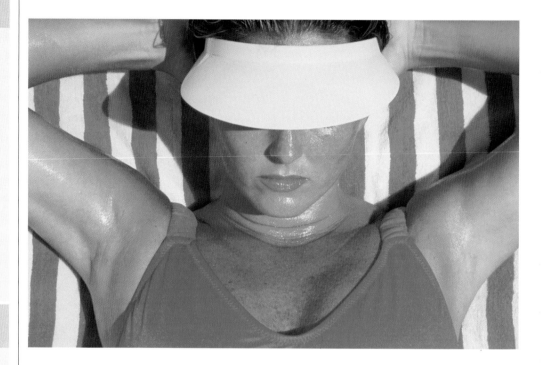

▲ *Sunstroke is often caused by lengthy exposure to the sun's heat. Someone who is unused to the heat, such as a person from a cold climate who goes to a hot climate and spends long hours sunbathing, is more at risk than a person who lives in a hot climate.*

Most people are used to thinking of the extremely serious heat disorder called sunstroke as something that happens only to people who stay out too long in the hot sun. However, the real cause of the condition is not the sun's rays but the intense heat that the sun produces. For this reason, doctors prefer to talk about heatstroke rather than sunstroke.

Any environment that gets hot can be dangerous. For instance, people who find themselves in very hot places such as engine rooms and steelworks can suffer the severe effects of sunstroke without ever being exposed to the sun.

## The body's reaction to heat

The body has two main mechanisms for losing heat. First, the blood vessels to the skin are dilated so that more blood flows to the surface, allowing it to lose heat through the skin into the air. Second, the sweat glands pour out salty fluid onto the surface of the skin, where it evaporates and heat is lost by the latent heat of vaporization (see Glands; Salt). It takes more than 500 times the amount of heat to turn 0.04 ounce (1 gr) of water 1.8°F (1°C) into vapor.

## Overheating

There are many ways in which the environment can intensify the effects of heat on the body. It is not, therefore, just a question of reading the degrees on the thermometer. If the air is humid, then this reduces the ease with which the sweat evaporates, so that it becomes more difficult to lose heat. Similarly, if the air is very still, less heat is lost from the surface of the body by convection.

People doing hard physical work in a hot environment are, of course, producing a lot of heat of their own. They may be losing up to 1 quart (0.9 l) of sweat every hour, compared with the

1 quart (0.9 l) per day of the sedentary worker in a temperate climate. This loss of salt and water can contribute to a condition known as heat exhaustion, which, unless checked, can lead to the eventual breakdown of the body's temperature-regulating mechanisms (see Temperature). However, as the body gets used to working in a hot environment, it adapts, and the loss of salts decreases, making the body less vulnerable to heat disorders.

## Additional risk factors

The very young and the very aged are most at risk from heat disorders, and consequently from heatstroke. This is because their temperature-regulating mechanisms are not very efficient. And because of this deficiency, older people also tend to wear heavy clothes even on sunny days, thereby increasing the risk of overheating still further.

There are several other predisposing factors. People who are unused to heat, who are very overweight, who drink heavily, or who are suffering from a feverish illness may also be at a greater risk from heatstroke (see Alcoholism; Obesity).

## Symptoms and dangers

The three basic signs of heatstroke are: a high temperature (more than 106°F [41°C]); a total absence of sweating; and, most seriously, problems of the nervous system that may lead to coma. Disturbances of mood, disorientation, and headache, often accompanied by dizziness and difficulty in walking, all happen in the early stages of heatstroke until consciousness is lost.

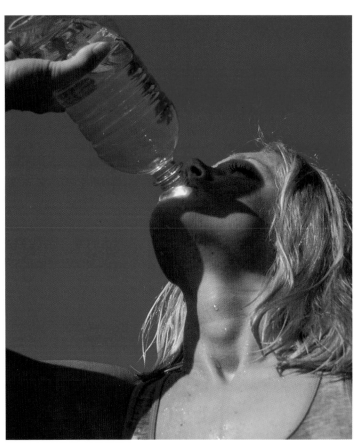

▲ *Drinking plenty of water in hot environments, especially if undergoing much physical exertion, helps prevent sunstroke.*

Fully developed heatstroke is an extremely dangerous condition and over 20 percent of sufferers may die, even with treatment. Even those who do recover may have persistent trouble in the nervous system and their balance and coordination may take months to return to normal. However, if treatment is prompt (at the first sign of symptoms and before consciousness is lost) then the chances of recovery are good.

## Treatment and prevention

As soon as any of the symptoms of heatstroke appear, it is essential to call a doctor immediately. Meanwhile, cool the patient down as quickly as possible. The temperature needs to be brought down to about 102°F (39°C), but no lower, as the patient's circulation may go into shock. Remove the patient's clothes and cover him or her with a thin cotton blanket, which should be continually doused in cold water. If possible, the best way to cool the patient down is in a tub of cold water. In a hospital, special slatted beds on which sufferers can be doused with water and cooled by fans are used.

The most sensible and effective way to fight sunstroke is, of course, prevention. This can be done simply by ensuring that the body is not overheated. This entails not staying out too long in the sun; wearing cool, loose clothing in the heat; and taking salt tablets and drinking plenty of liquids when doing physical work in very hot environments.

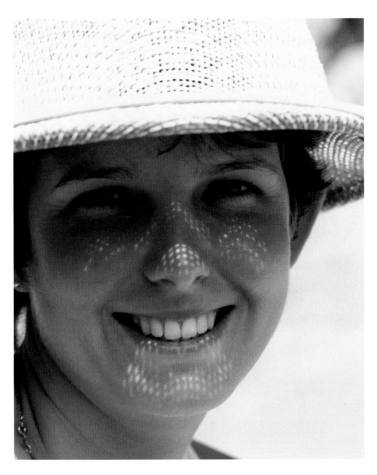

▲ *Wearing a hat, especially at midday when the sun is beating down directly, helps to keep the body from overheating.*

See also: **Heat and heat disorders; Perspiration; Prickly heat; Travel and health**

# Suppositories

**Can all medicines be taken in suppository form?**

No, and some drugs consisting of large complex molecules, such as vaccines and tissue extracts, cannot be given by mouth either. They have to be given by injection, since they will not go through the wall of the intestine into the bloodstream. The same principle applies in the rectum, and these types of drugs are useless if they are given by suppository. However, most drugs that we are used to taking by mouth in tablet or capsule form could be taken rectally in suppository form.

**Are there advantages to taking medication in suppository form?**

Yes, in certain circumstances there can be. A person who has an illness that involves vomiting may not be able to keep down drugs given by mouth, so an alternative route of administration must be found. Similarly, there are drugs that irritate the stomach, causing dyspepsia and vomiting. In this case, the suppository form may prove to be the best alternative.

**Are there any dangers in using suppositories?**

In general, no. Many people find their use distasteful, but it is rarely dangerous. Two points need to be borne in mind.

First, remember not to insert the suppository until you are sure that you are not going to want to use the toilet for some time.

Second, avoid getting into the habit of using suppositories regularly; people with hemorrhoids tend to do this. They are safe only if used for a short course. Prolonged use damages the tissues that line the rectum. In any case, if someone has troublesome hemorrhoids, he or she should visit the doctor, who will advise on treatment.

**Taking medicine by mouth or injection can sometimes be inappropriate for certain conditions. Introducing a drug rectally by means of suppositories is a safe and effective alternative.**

The term "suppository" describes a drug or medicine that is inserted into the rectum. This method offers an alternative to more traditional methods of taking medicines, such as by mouth (in the form of tablets, capsules, or liquid mixtures), by inhalation (in the form of gases or sprays), or by injection. Suppositories may also be inserted into the vagina when used in the treatment of vaginal infection; they are termed "pessaries."

Because of the way a suppository is used, it is made in a form that enables it to be used without undue discomfort. First, it is cone-shaped so that it can be pushed easily into the anus. Second, it is constructed from an oily or greasy base material so that it can be inserted without any difficulty or pain. The suppository slowly melts and the drug is gradually released, to be quickly absorbed by blood vessels in the rectal wall. There are often specific reasons why a drug should be administered by suppository rather than orally (as tablets or liquid), or by injection.

## HOW A SUPPOSITORY IS INSERTED

*With the patient in a comfortable position, here standing, the person inserting the suppository takes it in a gloved hand and gently pushes it into the rectum with one finger until the sphincter muscles grip on the finger's second joint. The suppository must be retained in the rectum as long as possible for it to be effective.*

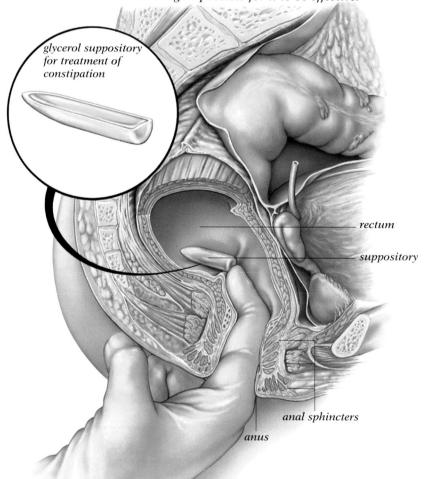

*glycerol suppository for treatment of constipation*

*rectum*

*suppository*

*anal sphincters*

*anus*

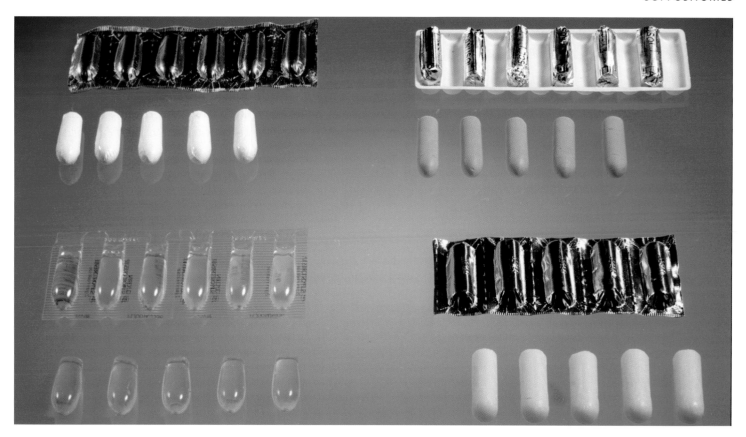

▲ *Suppositories are made in a pellet-shaped form. They are used to treat an extremely diverse range of conditions, from hemorrhoids to rheumatism.*

The most obvious reason for taking a medicine in suppository form is that the area the doctor wishes to treat is in the rectum or anus itself. Speedy and direct contact between the drug and an infection in this area can best be achieved by this method.

The use of suppositories may be preferred by both doctor and patient when a drug prescribed by the doctor causes stomach irritation. In addition, an unacceptable amount of indigestion may arise if the drug is taken in tablet form. Taking the drug by suppository avoids these side effects (see Side Effects).

Some drugs are broken down by gastric juices during their passage through the stomach and become useless. The suppository method will prevent this, since the drug is absorbed into the blood without going through the digestive process.

Drugs taken in suppository form are absorbed into the circulation more gradually than if taken by mouth, and sometimes this can be of positive benefit in treating some conditions. The release of the drug can be sustained over longer periods, perhaps lasting as long as 12 hours from a single dose. This method of drug administration also avoids the need to take tablets at frequent intervals, or to wake up during the night to take medication. When vomiting is a feature of an illness, it is not possible to give medicines by mouth, but taking drugs by suppository through the anal canal is ideal.

## Conditions treated

Suppositories are most commonly used in the treatment of hemorrhoids, and a great variety of suppositories are suitable for this purpose (see Hemorrhoids). Some contain astringents such as hammamelis or bismuth subgallate, which have the effect of shrinking the hemorrhoids; some are local anesthetics to diminish soreness; others contain mild antiseptics to prevent infection.

Suppositories are widely used in the treatment of constipation (see Constipation), especially in older people, because they go straight to the site where treatment is required. Glycerol suppositories (which generally contain 70 percent glycerol) soften and lubricate the feces, and are particularly useful if evacuation is painful. Bisacodyl and danthron suppositories are more powerful than glycerol and act by irritating the rectum into action.

Hydrocortisone suppositories are used on local inflammatory conditions of the anus and rectum, and nystatin suppositories are used for the treatment of thrush. Some rheumatic and arthritic conditions can also be treated with suppositories, usually when the drugs used (such as indomethacin and phenylbutazone) may cause side effects in the stomach if taken by mouth. The drug is absorbed just as effectively in the rectum as in the stomach but the side effects are avoided.

In some cases, respiratory disorders, pain (see Pain Management), and even vertigo are treated with drugs given by suppository. This is because some of the drugs used are most effective when absorbed slowly into the bloodstream.

Young children should not be given a suppository unless it is recommended by a doctor, although doctors sometimes give suppositories to babies. Long-term or habitual use of suppositories should also be avoided, as constant exposure to the chemicals in the suppositories could damage the tissues lining the rectum.

*See also:* **Anus; Arthritis; Lung and lung diseases; Pain; Rectum; Rheumatism; Thrush; Vagina; Vertigo; Vomiting**

# Surgery

## Questions and Answers

**What is the average length of an operation?**

Operations can last from a few minutes to many hours, sometimes as many as 10 or 12 hours. On average, abdominal surgery, such as a removal of the gallbladder, can take between one and three hours, depending on how straightforward the procedure is.

**My father has to have surgery on his bladder. His chest is bad so he will have spinal anesthesia. Will the surgery be painful?**

No. Spinal anesthesia should take away all painful sensation from the lower half of the body, and lasts for a few hours after surgery. During surgery, even though he will be awake he will be given a tranquilizing injection.

**How many years does it take to become a fully qualified surgeon?**

All surgeons have to go through a basic training to become a doctor, and this takes a minimum of four years. They then spend a year as an intern, after which they begin specialist jobs while working for their examinations for the American Board of Surgery. This usually takes a further four or five years, after which the surgeon in training carries on as a resident for five to seven years.

**Why do some patients have a tube inserted in their nose after they have undergone surgery?**

A nasogastric tube is passed through the nose into the stomach to remove secretions from the stomach before they build up, and is commonly used after surgery on the abdomen. The tube is left in place for two or three days until the intestines are able to work normally again.

**Surgical knowledge and techniques are continually advancing; keyhole surgery and endoscopy have resulted in faster recovery times and less invasive procedures; diagnostic imaging techniques help surgical accuracy.**

Surgery has evolved greatly in the past 100 years or so with technological advances that are of benefit to both patient and surgeon.

Until about a century ago, surgery was performed with no anesthesia (see Anesthetics) and with little regard for the problems of infection. As a result, some patients died directly as a result of the surgery rather than of the condition for which they were being treated.

Four major advances have revolutionized surgical procedures: anesthesia, asepsis, microsurgery, and minimally invasive (keyhole) surgery.

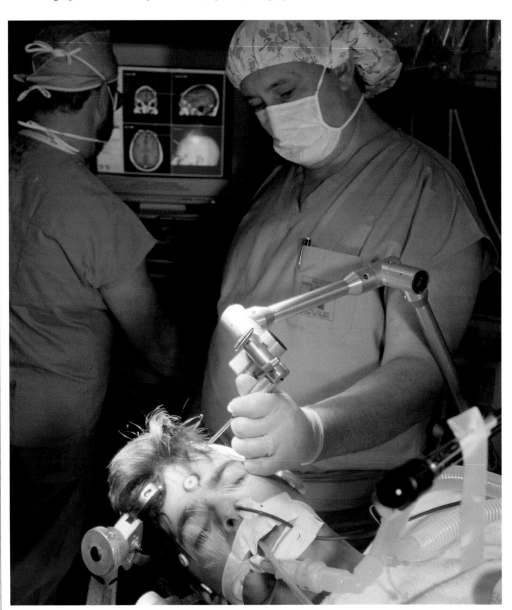

▲ *At a hospital in Chicago, a doctor drills into the head of a 21-year old patient who is undergoing brain surgery.*

## Anesthesia

In modern surgery, operations can be performed under local, regional, spinal, or general anesthesia. In local anesthesia, a solution of a drug (usually lignocaine) is injected into the tissues to be operated on. The effect is almost instantaneous and should provide complete anesthesia so that the patient cannot feel any pain at all. If pain is felt, it is because the drug was not injected into the right place. The effect of the anesthesia usually lasts for a few hours after the injection has been administered (see Anesthetics).

Regional anesthesia involves the use of the same drug, lignocaine, but in such a way that a whole region of the body is anesthetized. This can be achieved by injecting into or around a large nerve, or by putting a tourniquet around a limb and injecting the drug into a vein in the limb, thus filling up the blood vessels of the limb with the local anesthetic. Many operations can be performed using this type of anesthesia.

Spinal anesthesia is a method of blocking the pain impulses as they pass up the nerve column of the spine to the brain. This can be done in one of two ways, both of which involve passing a needle or a fine tube between two of the bones of the spine (the vertebrae). A local anesthetic drug can be injected into the fluid that surrounds the spinal cord (the cerebrospinal fluid), or it can be injected into the potential space outside the outer membrane, the dura mater, which sheaths the cord. The latter is a difficult technique known as epidural anesthesia, and calls for expertise and care. Spinal anesthetics do not involve loss of consciousness and are extensively used for surgery on the lower part of the body in patients in whom general anesthesia might involve some risk.

General anesthesia, which induces unconsciousness, involves the administration of drugs by injection and the inhalation of anesthetic gases. When this method is used, the patient is both insensitive to pain and also immobile. If necessary the patient can be paralyzed, so that the muscles throughout the body become lax, and this makes operating on the abdomen much easier. With the development of safer anesthetics, and safer anesthetic techniques, the surgeon can perform the operation without time constraints.

One of the improvements that went hand-in-hand with anesthetic technique was the realization, only about 50 years ago, that the transfusion of blood and saline during and after surgery greatly improves a patient's progress toward recovery.

## Aseptic techniques

In the 19th century, the discovery by the French medical pioneer Louis Pasteur that disease could be transmitted by organisms called bacteria paved the way for the development by the British surgeon Joseph Lister of aseptic techniques. Before this, surgery was performed in a large room before an audience (hence the British term "operating theater") by a surgeon who often took off his coat and put on another one covered with old blood. He did not wear rubber gloves, and the instruments were superficially clean, but they were not sterilized. Not surprisingly, all surgical wounds became infected. Joseph Lister found that spraying carbolic acid on and around the wound at the time of surgery decreased the incidence of infection. This technique, which was really an antiseptic technique, then led to aseptic techniques, in which bacteria were not allowed near the wound.

In modern surgery all equipment is sterilized, from the surgical instruments and suture materials to the surgeon's gloves and gown. The open wound is thus not contaminated, or contaminated very little, by extraneous bacteria. This technique has led to a near-zero rate of infection in so-called clean surgery such as hernia repairs (see Hernia). There is still a significant infection rate in dirty surgery, in which there is contamination with bacteria from within the patient. Examples of dirty surgery are removal of the appendix, or operations

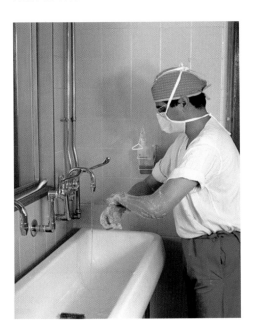

▼ *Although gloves are worn, a surgeon's skin must be scrupulously clean. He or she first scrubs with soap and water and then with an antiseptic such as iodine.*

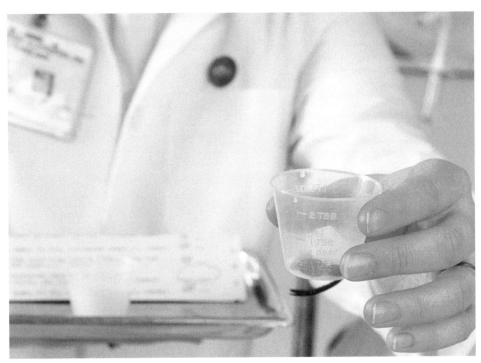

▼ *A nurse will check the patient's identity an hour or two prior to surgery, and will then administer the premedication, which prepares the patient for anesthesia.*

## Questions and Answers

**My mother had a tumor removed from her large intestine. When will we know whether the operation has been successful?**

Assuming she makes an uncomplicated recovery from the surgery, it will be one or two years before you will know whether the operation has been a success. The surgeon who performed the operation may be able to tell you more when he or she has a pathology report on the specimen. In any case, your mother will have to continue to be seen by the surgeon for several years to come.

**What are the risks involved in having major surgery today?**

This is very difficult to gauge, since there are so many factors involved. These include the age of the patient, the disease for which the surgery is being performed, and any other illnesses that the patient might have. In general, however, major surgery is undertaken only when the risks of not having the operation outweigh the risks of having it.

**I underwent surgery about a month ago and my operation scar still looks very red and prominent, although I was told by the doctor that it would not be noticeable. How long does it usually take before a surgical scar becomes less unsightly?**

Most surgical scars become red at about this stage, and do look ugly. However, given time, the redness disappears and by the end of a year the scar should be pale and faded. It may even continue to improve after a year, and so you shouldn't worry about it unless it is still prominent 18 months after surgery, in which case you should go back to your doctor. Unfortunately, there is really nothing that can be done to speed up this natural healing process. Try to be patient, and in time your scar should disappear or at least fade significantly so that you do not notice it.

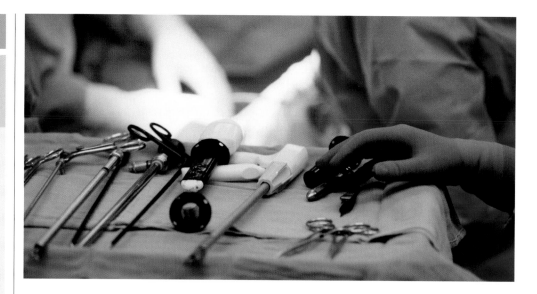

▲ *A selection of sterilized surgical instruments, appropriate for the surgical procedure to be performed, is ready for use in an operating theater.*

on the intestine. However, even with dirty operations, the use of modern antibiotics (see Antibiotics) is bringing down the infection rate significantly.

### Surgical stitches

There are various types of suture material in use today, each with its own special properties. Stitches can be divided into those that dissolve in the body tissues and those that stay permanently in the tissues, or are removed sometime after the operation. In the first category are catgut, collagen, and Dexon. Catgut is not, as the name suggests, made from cats' intestines, but is in fact made from the lining of sheep's intestines. The material is dried and twisted, and may be subject to a process similar to tanning to make it last longer in the tissues. It is then sterilized and packed in hermetically sealed tinfoil packs in alcohol. Dexon is a synthetic material that also dissolves in the tissues, but is not as pliable or as easy to knot as catgut during the stitching process.

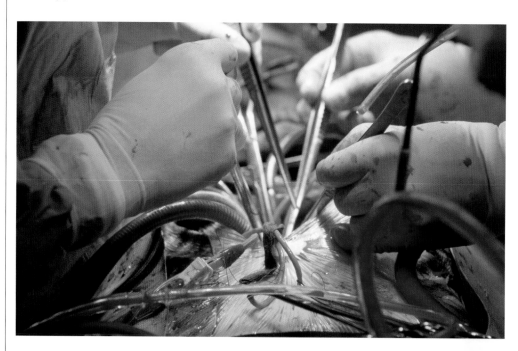

▼ *In this operation, a "Ross switch" is being performed, in which a patient's healthy heart valve is used to replace a faulty valve.*

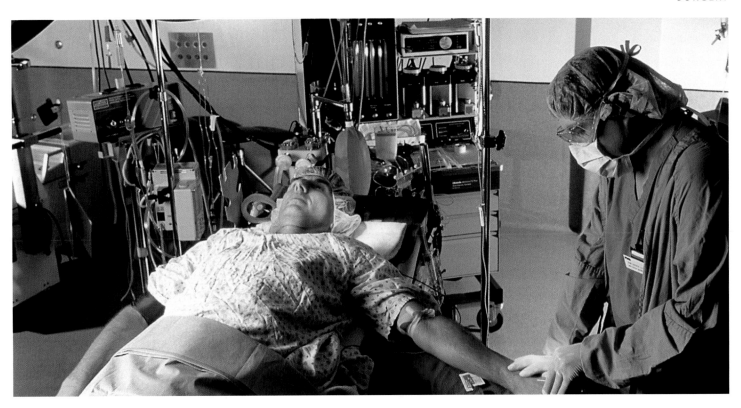

Among the stitches that are nonabsorbable are silk and linen thread, monofilament nylon, braided nylon, and wire. All these materials are used for specific purposes and are left in the body. They may weaken over the years, but it is possible to find traces of them in a patient many years later.

All these substances are used for tying around structures, when they are known as ligatures; and for stitching tissues together, when they are known as sutures (see Sutures). When sutures are used, the thread is fixed to the needle by the manufacturer by a process known as swaging. In this case the blunt end of the needle does not

*▲ Today's anesthesiologist has a wealth of equipment at hand. During surgery, he or she monitors the patient's heartbeat, measures blood pressure, and administers the anesthetic gases.*

have an eye, like a dressmaker's needle, but instead has a hollow end. The thread is pushed into the hollow end and the metal of the needle is pinched onto the thread. Thus when the needle is pulled through the tissue, no injury is caused by the knot of thread. There are different varieties of needle: some are made straight, to be handheld; some are curved, to be held in a special needle holder. The point of the needle may be conical, or it may be triangular in cross section so that it cuts through the tissue. This second type of needle is used for sewing up skin.

*▼ An operation in the early days of antiseptic surgery. The anesthetic used was chloroform, and the steam-operated carbolic spray, invented by Joseph Lister, produced an antiseptic atmosphere.*

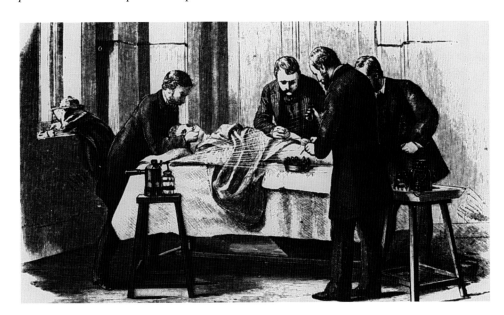

### Surgical instruments

With aseptic techniques and general anesthesia, there was a large advance in the techniques of operating, and many of the instruments used today were developed as far back as the end of the 19th century. There have been many modifications and new developments since, but the basic types of instrument have changed very little.

**Scalpels**: A modern surgical scalpel consists of a solid metal handle onto which can be clipped stainless steel blades of varying sizes. The blades are used only once, and several different blades may be used during the course of an operation. The essential feature of good surgical dissection

## Questions and Answers

**How does a surgeon decide if surgery is the best treatment?**

This varies according to the patient's condition. Some conditions, such as cancer of the colon, are best treated by surgery, and this would be performed unless the patient is otherwise unfit for surgery. A duodenal ulcer could be treated either by surgery or by medication, and the decision to operate depends on the patient's response to medical treatment or the likelihood of complications from the ulcer if surgery were not performed.

**I am very frightened of needles, and wonder if I will have to have an IV after I have my appendix removed. Could I do without one?**

It would be unwise, even dangerous to have any kind of major surgery without an IV line that gives an anesthetist quick access to the circulating blood. Anesthesia is nearly always induced intravenously, and it is routine to establish an IV line before starting. It is an almost painless procedure; you need not watch, and you will feel only a slight prick on your hand.

**My husband had surgery on his stomach a few days ago and is terribly worried that he might burst the stitches by coughing or moving about. Is this possible?**

No. The materials used to stitch the abdominal wall are extremely strong, and it is very unlikely that a bout of coughing would cause them to break.

**Is the catgut that surgeons use for stitches really made from cats' intestines?**

No, it is not real catgut. It is made from the lining of sheep's intestines, and is the same material used for the strings of musical instruments. However, the surgical variety is treated so that it is free from bacteria. Buried surgical catgut usually takes about two months to absorb completely.

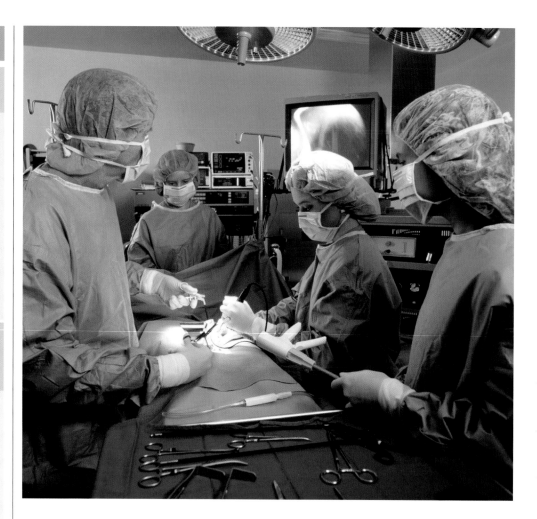

▲ *A surgical procedure called laparoscopy is being performed, in which a viewing instrument, a laparoscope, is used to look at the interior of the abdomen.*

is that the tissues should be cut cleanly, and so it is always necessary to have a sharp scalpel blade. As well as differing in size, scalpels also differ in shape to suit varying kinds of surgery.

**Scissors**: There are many different designs of scissors—some long, some short, some curved, and some straight. They are always of the finest-quality steel, and they are kept in excellent working order. Many surgeons have their own favorite design of scissors.

**Artery forceps**: If an artery or a vein is cut during the course of surgery, it is first clipped with artery forceps in two places, and the vessel is cut between the two forceps. Artery forceps look a little like scissors at first glance, but are really a pair of tiny pincers, with a ratchet mechanism on the handle so that they stay shut at a particular tension. There are dozens of different designs of artery forceps, differing only slightly in size and shape.

**Retractors**: These are specially shaped pieces of metal that are used to hold the edges of an incision wound open during an operation. They can be held by an assistant, or are designed to be self-retaining; that is, they are attached to a frame so that they can be fixed into the wound at a predetermined distance apart. Surgery on the abdomen would be impossible without retraction.

As well as all the instruments described, there are countless others that are used for various specialist procedures. In a modern operating room, there are various packs made up containing all the instruments that might be needed for a specific operation. The pack is labeled on the outside, and always has the same numbers and types of instrument for a particular procedure. As a result, some instruments are repeatedly sterilized and are not used, but the system ensures that time is not wasted during surgery. If an unexpected surgical procedure has to be undertaken during the course of another operation, then extra instruments can be brought in. At the end of surgery, all the instruments that have actually been used are cleansed and put back in the tray with the unused instruments. The whole tray is then checked carefully before being wrapped up, labeled, and sterilized ready for the next time. A large modern hospital has many

## Surgeons: Who they are

| TITLE OF SPECIALTY | WHAT THEY OPERATE ON |
| --- | --- |
| Neurological surgeon | Brain and spinal cord |
| Ear, nose, and throat surgeon | Nose, tonsils, adenoids, tongue, face, ears, larynx, thyroid gland, upper part of esophagus, floor of mouth |
| Ophthalmic surgeon | Eyes, eyelids, and tear ducts |
| Orthopedic surgeon | Bones (except the bones of the skull) |
| Obstetrician and gynecologist | Uterus, ovaries, vagina, and cesarean births |
| Thoracic surgeon | Heart, lungs, esophagus, diaphragm, chest wall |
| Pediatric surgeon | Babies and small children |
| Urologist | Kidneys, ureters, bladder, urethra, prostate gland |
| General surgeon | Stomach, gallbladder, liver, intestines, appendix, breasts, thyroid, glands in face (salivary glands), main arteries and veins, lumps under the skin, hernias, and hemorrhoids |

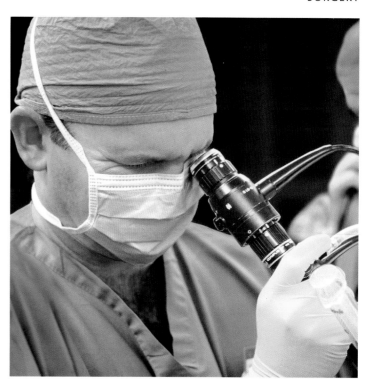

▲ *A doctor looks through a bronchoscope at the bronchi (airways) in the lungs. The instrument is used to help diagnose lung diseases such as cancer and tuberculosis.*

duplicate sets of instruments so that several operations can be performed on the same day without having to wait for the instruments to be sterilized again.

### Microsurgery

The use of an operating microscope, from the 1960s onward, was the third major revolution in surgery. These binocular instruments were introduced first by ophthalmic surgeons and were then taken up by otologists. They allowed a remarkable degree of delicacy and precision so that operations previously impossible soon became routine. Microsurgery rapidly highlighted the relative crudeness of current operating instruments, and a succession of generations of ever more delicate, miniaturized, and refined tools were developed specially for use under a microscope. Soon surgeons in other disciplines exploited microsurgery and it gradually extended its scope to other areas in which magnification was essential. Vascular surgeons, concerned with repair to small blood vessels; neurological surgeons joining cut nerves; and gynecologists working on fallopian tubes and suspected cancer of the cervix all found that the scope of their practice could be greatly extended by microsurgery. One of the advances allowed by this technique is the successful reattachment of limbs that have been severed in accidents. This involves rejoining arteries, veins, nerves, tendons, and muscles (see Microsurgery).

### Minimally invasive surgery

Experience has shown that the factor mainly responsible for the length of the recovery period after surgery is the time taken for a long incision to heal. Surgical incisions involve not only skin, but also muscle and various tissue planes under the skin. The development of fiber-optic and other forms of internal viewing instruments (endoscopes) made it possible for the interior of the body to be examined either through natural orifices or through a tiny surgical opening. Surgeons then found that it was easy to take small samples (biopsies) for pathological examination with a small knife attached to the endoscopes. The next step was endoscopic instruments to perform surgical procedures other than cutting.

When it became apparent that a range of surgical operations could be done through two or three ports—short metal or plastic tubes less than half an inch across—the fourth surgical revolution was under way. Ports involve tiny incisions and small splits in the muscle layers. Often these require only one or two stitches. Gases are blown in to make space; then miniaturized, closed-circuit television cameras can be used via fiber-optic channels. Instruments can be operated by remote control while the surgeon sits comfortably watching his or her progress on a TV monitor. It is even possible for a surgeon in New York to perform an operation on a patient in London. After this kind of surgery, patients can often return to full activity the following day.

### The surgeon

The person who performs operations is a surgeon. He or she is a qualified doctor who then has further specialist training, but this was not always so. At one time, surgeons were members of the Worshipful Company of Barber-Surgeons—that is, they were barbers who also dabbled in a bit of surgery. Presumably they were adept at using a sharp instrument. The barber's pole, with its red and white stripes, is supposed to be a symbol of blood and a bandage.

After qualifying as a doctor, a person who wants to become a surgeon has to pass further exams to become fully qualified. He or she takes these examinations in separate parts over a period of about five years after qualifying, and while working as an apprentice surgeon. During this time, the surgeon learns to perform operations himself or herself, being taught by an experienced senior surgeon.

People often wonder how a training surgeon gets to do his or her first operation. It is a gradual process, starting with very small surgical procedures under strict supervision, and building up to more major surgery. By the time a trainee surgeon performs a major operation, he or she has probably helped the senior surgeon with the same type of operation many times.

### What the job entails

A surgeon's job entails seeing patients, examining them, diagnosing the cause of their symptoms, and then deciding whether or not the condition is best treated with medication or by surgery. If the surgeon decides to treat the patient with medication, the surgeon may undertake this task, or may ask a physician (a medical specialist who treats illnesses with drugs) to see the patient and take over the case. If he or she decides that surgery is appropriate, then the relevant procedure will be performed.

It may be that at the time of the operation there are several options and the surgeon will have to decide which is the most suitable operation to perform in light of what he or she knows about the patient and the illness. After the operation, the surgeon will see the patient on the ward and

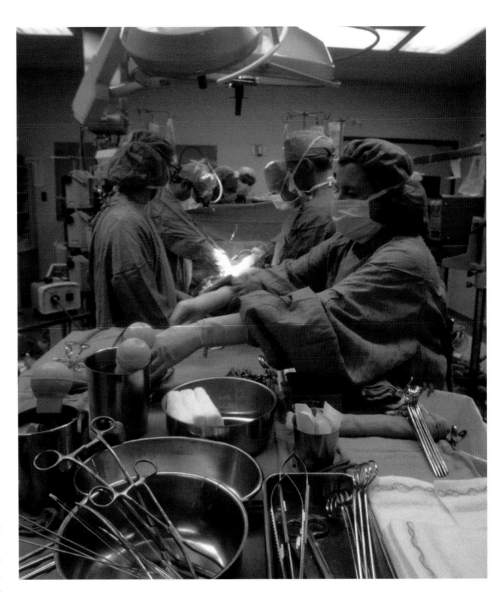

▲ *All the equipment used in surgery must be accounted for after the operation— even the swabs. These absorbent pads, which are used to keep the operating site free from blood, are hung up and counted.*

deal with any complications, should they arise. He or she will also be responsible for seeing patients on follow-up visits until it is felt that they are well enough to be discharged back into the care of their own physicians. The contemporary surgeon, therefore, may be considerably involved in the care of the patient, both before and after the operation. In fact, he or she probably spends only about one-third of the work time actually working in the operating room.

### Different types of surgery

There are hundreds of different operations that are done on the human body; in general they fall into eight broad groups. They are: repair operations on hernias, fractured bones, or parts of the body that have suffered injury; removal of tumors, ulcers, limbs, and overactive glands; division of strictures, such as releasing tight fibrous bands pressing on a nerve; transplantation of organs; insertion of prostheses such as breast implants and heart valves; bypassing blocked arteries; correction of congenital deformities; and skin grafts.

Surgical operations can go wrong; there may be damage to other structures near the operative site, bleeding, infection, or poor wound healing. However, with improved skills and technology these risks have been greatly reduced.

### Specialties

Surgeons are divided into groups of specialists such as neurological; ear, nose, and throat; ophthalmic; orthopedic; obstetric; thoracic; pediatric; and urological. Each surgeon has his or her own territory, except for a general surgeon, who is trained to do a wide range of operations covering many areas of the body. Most general surgeons, however, also tend to be specialists within one smaller field.

Most hospitals have at least one general surgeon, but not every hospital has all the other specialists, so the general surgeon may often be called on to perform a wide range of operations in an emergency.

*See also:* **Bacteria; Infection and infectious diseases**

# Surrogacy

**How much will a couple usually have to pay to arrange to have a child by a surrogate mother?**

If the couple get a surrogate mother through an agency (now the normal route) they can expect to pay around $35,000: $10,000 to $12,000 of that typically goes to the surrogate mother; $15,000 to legal expenses; and at least $10,000 to agency fees. Additional fees for the carrier's prenatal care and delivery will be required if these are not covered by insurance.

**What are some of the features of a typical surrogate contract?**

A typical surrogate contract requires the surrogate to agree to be inseminated with sperm provided by the man whose wife is sterile, to carry the child conceived to term, and to surrender the child to the couple for adoption immediately after delivery. The couple would be required to pay the surrogate's medical bills and a specified fee for her services, and to take the child whether or not it has any mental or physical defects. Sometimes the surrogate mother is required to undergo amniocentesis and to abort the fetus if the results show any abnormality.

**Why would a woman want to go through pregnancy and the pain of labor to have someone else's baby?**

Some surrogate mothers say they enjoy being pregnant and look forward to being pregnant without the responsibility of raising another child. Others have had an abortion or a miscarriage, or have had a loss in their lives and feel a need to resolve it by bearing a child, even if it is for someone else. Some do it out of the desire to help a couple have the baby they could not have by themselves. Some women may do it just for the money. This last motive is the one that has given the most concern.

**Surrogacy is surrogate motherhood; that is, a woman becomes pregnant by surgical implantation of a fertilized egg or by artificial insemination, and gives birth to a baby for an infertile couple.**

Surrogate motherhood is fast becoming one of the thorniest controversies of modern family law. The technical aspects of maternal surrogacy involve major arguments between those who favor this arrangement and those who do not.

## The types of surrogacy

The term "surrogate mother" was first used in connection with a very sophisticated medical procedure called in vitro fertilization (IVF) and embryo transfer. This technique was first employed in the late 1970s in situations where both prospective parents were fertile but an abnormality affecting the woman, such as blocked or missing fallopian tubes, prevented conception. In this procedure, an ovum is surgically removed from the woman, fertilized outside her body with her husband's sperm, and then transferred into the woman's uterus (see Ovaries; Sperm; Uterus).

However, some women are not able to bear a child. One out of every 1,000 women, for example, is born without a uterus, and a variation of the IVF-embryo transfer procedure is used to overcome the problem. The fertilized egg is transferred into the uterus of another woman, who then carries the pregnancy to term. In a most unusual surrogacy arrangement of this type, a 48-year-old woman gave birth to triplets in 1987. She was acting as a surrogate for her daughter, so the children she gave birth to were her genetic grandchildren (see Genetics).

The term "surrogate mother" is also applied to a different sort of maternal surrogacy arrangement known as artificial insemination. This procedure involves injecting semen into the vagina when an anatomic abnormality in the male prevents direct fertilization, or when the male is infertile (see Infertility). In the latter case, the sperm is usually provided by an anonymous donor. The child that is conceived is genetically linked to the inseminated woman but not to her husband.

The newest use of artificial insemination resulted in 65 births in 1986, and gave rise to the current meaning of the term "surrogate mother"—also now commonly referred to as a "gestational carrier." This method involves introducing the sperm of a man whose wife is infertile into a woman who has contracted to bear the child conceived as a result of the insemination, which is then given to the couple after the birth. The genetic father of the child is obviously the husband. There is no biological link, however, between the child and the wife.

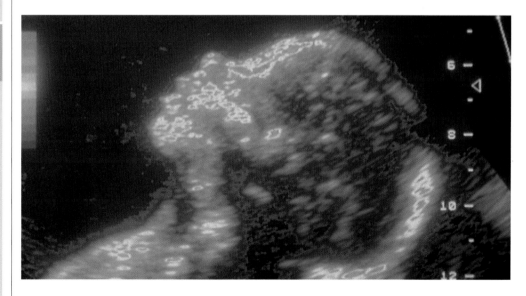

▲ *An ultrasound scan shows a clear profile of the head of a fetus at 22 gestational weeks.*

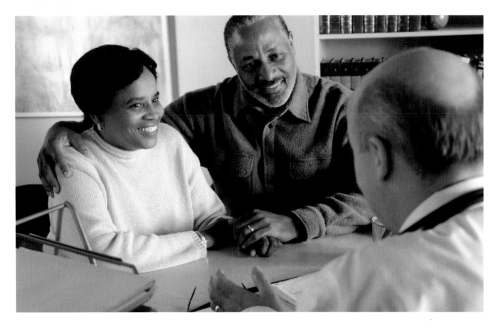

▲ *Once medical tests have revealed why a couple are unable to conceive, a doctor will advise other relevant options to them before he or she will suggest surrogacy.*

The whole issue of surrogate motherhood received national attention in 1986, when a surrogate mother, Mary Beth Whitehead, refused to surrender the daughter she had borne for Elizabeth Stern and Mrs. Stern's husband, William, with whose sperm she had been artificially inseminated. Mrs. Whitehead and the Sterns had been brought together by a private agency specializing in surrogate parenting arrangements. After a long and widely publicized trial, a judge ruled that the contract between Mrs. Whitehead and the Sterns was valid and assigned sole custody of the child to Mr. Stern. Mrs. Whitehead later won on appeal.

Another distressing case occurred in Britain in 1997. A nurse, age 31, had been paid $18,000 by a Dutch married couple and agreed to undergo artificial insemination with the husband's semen and to hand over the resulting baby at birth. The nurse had become pregnant, but in May 1997 informed the couple that she had aborted the baby (see Abortion). A few days later, however, she confessed that this was untrue and that she had lied because she wanted to keep the baby.

The case received wide publicity and acted as a focus for the expression of public opinion on the matter of surrogacy. As is inevitable in such matters, emotions were aroused and views were strongly polarized. One view expressed abhorrence at the idea of treating babies as commodities to be traded; the other was the view that women have the right to have children, whatever the means.

This case also prompted an editorial in the prestigious British medical journal *The Lancet*. In this, attention was drawn to Article 16 of the Universal Declaration of Human Rights issued by the General Assembly of the United Nations in 1948. The article states that: "Men and women of full age, without any limitation due to race, nationality, or religion, have the right to marry and to found a family."

Medical advances since 1948 have brought possibilities that could never have been considered by those who drafted this article, and the declaration has been interpreted as justifying all kinds of procreative methods. One of the consequences of such methods is, of course, surrogacy, with all its accompanying social and ethical problems.

*The Lancet*'s editorial makes the point strongly that "the rampant marketization of reproductive medicine demands urgent reassessment." There is criticism of the lack of leadership shown by the medical profession in calling for serious study of the reasons for these ethical shifts and evaluation of their likely consequences. "This shameful silence," it concludes, "leaves the market as the only voice to be heard, a voice that threatens to drown out those who raise even the most reasoned of objections."

## The arguments involved

The Catholic church, which opposes all forms of intervention that it feels sever procreation from the marital union, has stated that surrogate motherhood "offends the dignity and the right of the child to be conceived, carried in the womb, brought into the world, and brought up by its parents."

Other institutions and individuals object to any form of parental surrogacy on a variety of moral, ethical, and philosophical grounds.

However, it is surrogate motherhood arrangements like the one entered into by Mary Beth Whitehead and the Sterns that have galvanized advocates and opponents of surrogacy .

The advocates have argued that a surrogacy arrangement is the only hope for many couples of ever having a baby, and that a woman donating her ovum is really not all that different from the widely accepted practice of a man donating his sperm to a sperm bank.

Those who are opposed to surrogacy argue that anonymously donating sperm is a far cry from the woman's role of being artificially inseminated, bringing a pregnancy to term, giving birth, and then having to surrender the baby (see Birth).

Some people worry about the long-term effects of surrogacy on the surrogate mother. How many surrogate mothers will come to regret their decision the way Mary Beth Whitehead did? But champions of surrogate parenting contend that the great majority of surrogate mothers actually experience a sense of fulfillment from having helped a couple in need. They also suggest that women like Mary Beth Whitehead, who found she could not part with the child, would probably not become surrogate mothers in the first place if they were given better psychological counseling initially (see Counseling).

The antisurrogacy camp wonders about the adverse reactions children might have when they learn that their genetic mothers brought them into the world, probably for a fee, and then surrendered them. This camp also asks if these children will experience profound feelings of rejection and how their own future attitudes about having and raising children will be influenced. The prosurrogacy camp responds that these children would not exist were it not for the arrangement between the surrogate mother and the sperm donor, and that bringing children into the world in this way will soon be so common that surrogate-born children will not feel unusual.

In the light of these conflicting arguments, it would seem to be almost impossible to arrive at an ethical arrangement for surrogacy that does not simultaneously offend some people and interfere with the liberties or rights of others.

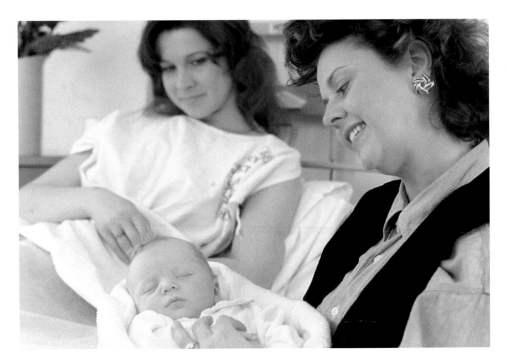

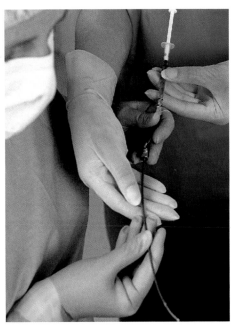

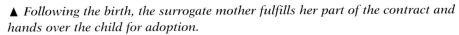

▲ *Following the birth, the surrogate mother fulfills her part of the contract and hands over the child for adoption.*

▲ *After in vitro fertilization, a catheter is used to transfer the healthy embryo into the mother's uterus via the cervix.*

Attempts to establish guidelines are likely to end in paradox. This is inevitable, since the central fact in surrogacy is the separation of gestation, with its emotional and emotive elements, from nurturing, rearing, and upbringing, which has its own emotional concomitants. This consequence of surrogacy, incidentally, highlights the extraordinary level of compassion shown by voluntary surrogate mothers in carrying and then donating the child, usually to a relative, without thought of personal gain. It is in striking contrast to the blatant consumerism of women who think they can use surrogacy as an easy way to earn a large sum of money. The experience of such women is likely to be a painful reminder to them that there are more important things than money.

### The need for legislation

The issues of human rights that are raised by surrogacy are so pressing that effective legislation to control the practice is essential. Under normal circumstances, the woman who bears the child is legally the mother, and her husband, if any, is legally the father. Surrogacy legislation cannot entirely ignore this principle, which is based not only on purely historical principles, but also on the recognition, or at least the strong presumption, that the woman who bears and delivers the child, even if it is genetically unrelated to her, has a greater psychological and legal claim on the child than anyone else.

Disputes over surrogacy have given rise to several custody cases and, in these, this principle has usually been upheld. It is not, however, universally held. Some research has shown that at least 40 percent of people may dispute it and opt for the genetic relationship. Many women take this view, although the view is even more prevalent among men.

The question of the rights of embryos to achieve existence as humans may also have to be considered by legislators. This has been held to be grounds for allowing surrogacy in cases in which a frozen embryo would otherwise be destroyed.

In 1989, in a case involving a frozen embryo, Judge Young found for the potential mother, Mary Sue Davies, holding that such an embryo should be defined as a "human being waiting to be born."

The argument against surrogate parenting arrangements that seems to have raised the most concern is that surrogate motherhood is little more than a formalized form of baby selling. No state, of course, permits a couple to sell a baby, and most states have statutes that forbid compensating a woman who offers her child for adoption.

The antisurrogacy forces say that states should pass bills that prohibit the payment of a fee that goes above and beyond medical expenses to any surrogate mother. They would also make illegal the fees paid to the agencies that make surrogacy arrangements.

Those in favor of surrogate parenting counter that it is not baby selling, because the father is genetically related to the child. Many women, they claim, would still be willing to act as surrogates even if fees were made illegal. Many state legislatures have passed bills that either strictly regulate surrogate parenting arrangements or make them entirely illegal.

Some permit the practice, but limit or prohibit the payment of fees to the surrogate mother or to any intermediaries. Most require psychological counseling for the prospective surrogate mother, legal representation for all parties, and court approval of the conditions set down in the contract.

While some legislation would require a surrogate mother to surrender the child to the father at the time of birth, other bills propose allowing the surrogate a specified period of time following the birth to decide if she still wants to give the child up. Whatever laws are passed, they will be tested in the courts, and the debate over surrogacy will no doubt be a matter of contention both in and outside of the courts for some time to come.

See also: **Artificial methods of conception; In vitro fertilization; Pregnancy**

# Sutures

## Questions and Answers

**Does it hurt to have skin stitches removed after surgery?**

No, not really. Modern materials used for stitches are much smoother than the old materials and slide easily through the tissues. It's really only the thought of having stitches taken out that makes it hurt. Remember it is the stitch that's being cut, not you.

**After major surgery do internal stitches last for a long time?**

Yes. Some of the stitch material used will last for a lifetime. Monofilament nylon, for instance, is almost inert and does not cause any tissue reaction. It will still be there in 30 years' time, although it may be weaker than it was when it was originally inserted.

**I recently had surgery on my stomach. How long will the stitches have to stay in?**

Usually between 7 and 10 days. If they are taken out before this time the wound may come apart; if they are left in longer an inflammation may develop around the area of the stitches.

**After abdominal surgery, is it possible to burst the stitches by coughing or straining?**

It would be very unusual. The strength of an abdominal wound closure depends on the internal stitches, not the stitches in the skin. Most surgeons therefore use a nonabsorbable material, such as nylon, to repair the muscle layers. Previously, catgut was used, but it lost strength so quickly that the wound could burst. Now, however, if the abdominal muscles have been stitched up satisfactorily with the kind of thread that lasts indefinitely, the stitches should be able to bear the strain of repeated coughing.

**Sutures are simply surgical stitches. They are an efficient method of keeping a wound closed while the tissues heal. Sutures are made in a variety of materials and can be absorbable or nonabsorbable.**

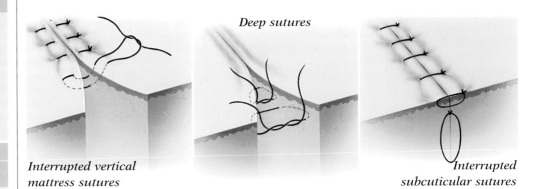

*Deep sutures*

*Interrupted vertical mattress sutures*

*Interrupted subcuticular sutures*

▲ *The interrupted vertical mattress and subcuticular stitches are those most commonly used. The latter eliminates any scarring from holes made by the needles. Deep sutures are used with other stitches when there would be a gap, or dead space, beneath the surface. With all three kinds, however, each stitch is individually tied, so that if one gives way, the others remain secure, unlike in continuous stitching. The actual choice is dictated by the surgeon's preference, and by practicalities such as tissue type, location, and final cosmetic appearance.*

When a surgeon stitches tissues back together he or she may use stitches that are very similar to those used by a tailor or dressmaker. The materials used can be divided into two basic types: those that dissolve over a period of time, and those that last for a lifetime. The former include catgut and Dexon, a synthetic substance; the latter include nylon, silk, linen, and wire.

## Methods and materials

The two edges of a wound may be stitched together in different ways. A continuous stitch may be used with a knot at each end, or the same effect can be obtained by inserting a row of separate stitches, each with its own knot. Using separate stitches (interrupted sutures) ensures that if one knot comes undone, or the material used breaks, the whole seam will not come apart. The decision whether or not to use absorbable stitches depends on many factors, the most important being the speed at which the tissues are likely to heal. Dissolvable sutures lose their strength early and so are used when healing occurs quickly, as in stomach repair surgery, when the wound will heal in a few days (see Healing). By contrast, for a hernia repair, most surgeons use nylon stitches, which remain strong for many years, and especially until scar tissue has formed. If absorbable sutures were used, the hernia would be more likely to recur.

## Skin stitches

There are many ways of joining skin. Continuous or interrupted stitches may be used, with absorbable or nonabsorbable materials. Metal clips or staples may be used, or butterflies made of adhesive tape. When nonabsorbable sutures are chosen, they are usually nylon or silk, and are left in the skin for about a week, until the wound is healed enough so that it will not reopen.

Sutures on the face are usually removed after a few days because the skin heals quickly, and because, if they are left in position too long, they will leave puncture marks. Absorbable sutures, usually inserted as one continuous thread just under the skin, cannot be seen from the outside.

*See also:* **Hernia; Plastic and reconstructive surgery; Scars; Surgery**

# Swellings

**A swelling is usually just a simple and passing reaction to infection or injury. It should not be ignored, however, since it can also be a symptom of an underlying condition that may require prompt medical treatment.**

Swellings can be found in any part of the body, in the skin or in the structures that lie beneath it. There are many causes of swellings, ranging from a boil beneath the skin to a swelling caused by a strain or sprain of a joint.

## Infections and injuries

Swellings are caused by many different conditions. Infected areas become filled with blood in an attempt to get rid of the invading bacteria or viruses. An infected finger is a good example; it becomes obviously swollen, red, hot, and painful. Swelling also occurs as a result of injury, and has the effect of cushioning the injured part and protecting it until it has had time to heal. This

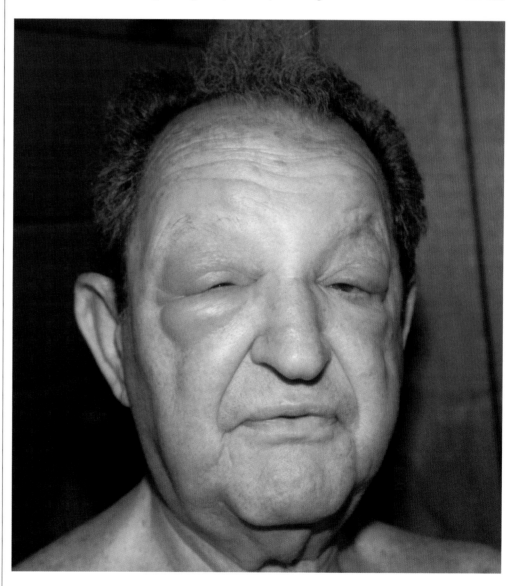

▲ *Bites and stings can cause extreme swelling; as is the case with this man—four hours after being bitten near the eye by a hornet.*

## Questions and Answers

**My four-year-old son has swollen neck glands all the time. Why?**

Children have large lymph glands and tonsils to deal with new virus infections with which they are in contact. The glands swell in response to various infections such as tonsillitis and return to their normal size when the infection has been overcome, but infections may be prolonged.

**Why does an ankle swell so much if it is sprained?**

When you walk, your weight is transferred from one foot to the other. A minor twist of the ankle when it is bearing a body's weight can result in severe damage to the ligaments that support it. Fluid leaks from the tiny damaged blood vessels into the tissues around the ankle. There may or may not be obvious bruising. The swelling can be reduced by using ice to constrict the blood vessels, elevation, and compression with an elasticized bandage. NSAIDs will control pain and inflammation.

**Why do some people's feet swell on long air journeys?**

Normally, blood is helped back to the heart from the feet by muscles that squeeze the veins when a person is walking. Sitting for long periods with the feet down does not improve the return of blood to the heart. The atmospheric pressure in an airplane is usually low; all these factors allow fluid to escape from the veins into the tissues of the feet. This makes the feet swell.

**Why do my face and tongue swell when I eat shellfish?**

You are allergic to shellfish. Swelling caused by allergy is known as angioneurotic edema. Never eat shellfish, and ask what is in food you have not prepared yourself.

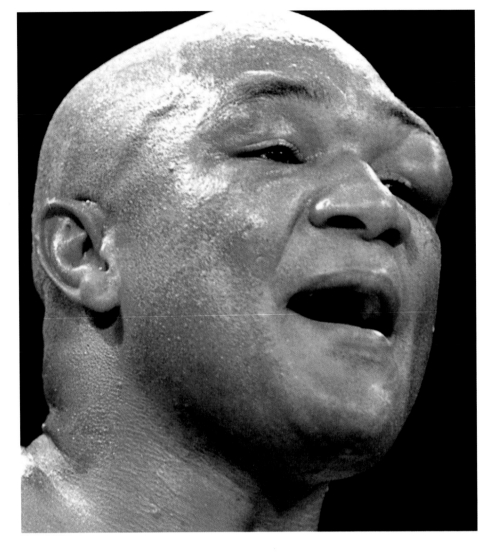

## Get medical advice if you have these symptoms

If you have a new ankle swelling and symptoms such as shortness of breath, chest pain, or fatigue.

If you have a very swollen, painful joint. If you know you have injured the joint, apply a firm elasticized bandage and take painkillers and rest it as much as possible. The swelling should disappear in a few days; if not see your doctor.

If you would like a skin lump removed for cosmetic reasons, or if you are worried about it.

If you have an infection in the skin that is more than a small boil.

If you swell up in response to an allergic substance.

If you have a growing swelling and you don't know what it is.

If you have a swollen abdomen that you don't think is due to being overweight or being constipated or having poor muscle strength.

If you notice a breast lump.

If you have a hernia.

▲ *Various swellings on the face are an occupational hazard in the world of boxing, as George Foreman displays.*

is often seen in a joint, such as the knee or ankle joint. If the injury is serious, the joint becomes filled with fluid made up of an increase in the normal synovial fluid found inside every joint, and fluid that leaks from torn capillary blood vessels and lymphatic vessels.

## Edema

Swollen ankles are caused by fluid that leaks from the small blood vessels of the lower legs and is not returned efficiently into the blood system to be pumped around the body. If the swelling is pressed firmly with the thumb, then the fluid is squeezed out from under the thumb, leaving a depression in the tissues. This swelling is called edema (see Edema). Mild edema is very common, and people who are overweight are more prone to ankle swelling. Women often notice that their ankles swell just before a period. Contraceptive pills may make this condition worse (see Contraception).

The ankles also have a tendency to swell during pregnancy, partly because of the increased pressure of the baby on the large veins in the pelvis. Very swollen ankles, however, may be a sign of toxemia of pregnancy and should never be ignored. Some pregnant women may also find that their hands and faces swell a little (see Preeclampsia; Pregnancy).

Puffiness of the face, especially around the eyes, is also a very common form of minor swelling that frequently occurs on waking. The exact cause is not known, but the swelling can be reduced by lying on the back instead of on the face, avoiding heavy night creams, and splashing the face with very cold water.

More persistent edema is often a symptom of an underlying condition. For example, even minor degrees of heart failure may produce ankle swelling. If the swelling is severe, medical advice should be sought, especially if there is shortness of breath.

Fluid also builds up in the body in a certain type of kidney disease called nephrotic edema, in liver disease, and if the person suffers from malnutrition. In all these cases there is a lack of protein in the blood, and water escapes into the tissues, producing swelling (see Kidneys and Kidney Diseases).

## Varicose veins and thrombosis

Varicose veins are also a common cause of swollen ankles (see Varicose Veins). Deep vein thrombosis in a vein in the calf can cause a swollen ankle and a swollen painful calf because of the obstruction of the blood flow by a clot. Wearing elastic support hose will help to reduce an ankle swelling, and the sufferer should elevate his or her legs and feet as often as possible. Diuretic tablets may be prescribed to reduce the edema (see Diuretics).

## Allergies

Sometimes people will swell up in just a few minutes if they are in contact with something they are allergic to, or if they have eaten something to which they are allergic. It is a frightening experience for the person concerned. Often the face is affected and the eyelids swell with fluid and may completely close the eyes. This condition of acute swelling caused by fluid in response to an allergic substance is called angioneurotic edema. The most common cause of this is probably an insect bite or sting (see Allergies).

Anyone who has ever suffered from this type of allergic condition should ask his or her doctor for advice and will probably have to carry antihistamine tablets in the event of such an allergic reaction.

## Skin swellings

Urticaria is a skin condition in which hard, white, itchy swellings quickly appear in the skin as a result of skin contact with an allergic substance. The skin is often the site for swellings, either from sebaceous cysts or from fatty lumps, known as lipomas. Both conditions are benign. Sebaceous cysts are often seen in young men, on the neck or upper chest or scalp. They cause few problems unless they become infected, but are often removed for cosmetic reasons. Lipomas may range in size from being just noticeable to being the

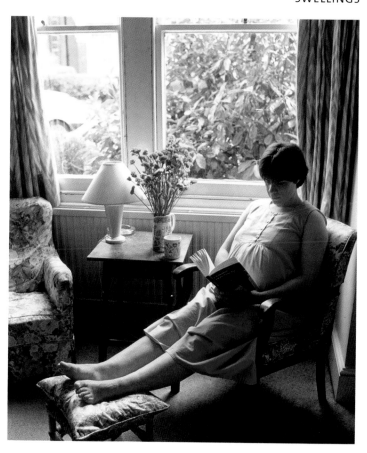

▲ *Ankles often swell during pregnancy. Resting with the legs raised will help keep discomfort to a minimum.*

▼ *Long air journeys in which travelers don't have the opportunity to move about often result in swollen feet and ankles. Always wear comfortable shoes or slippers and, if possible, keep your feet up.*

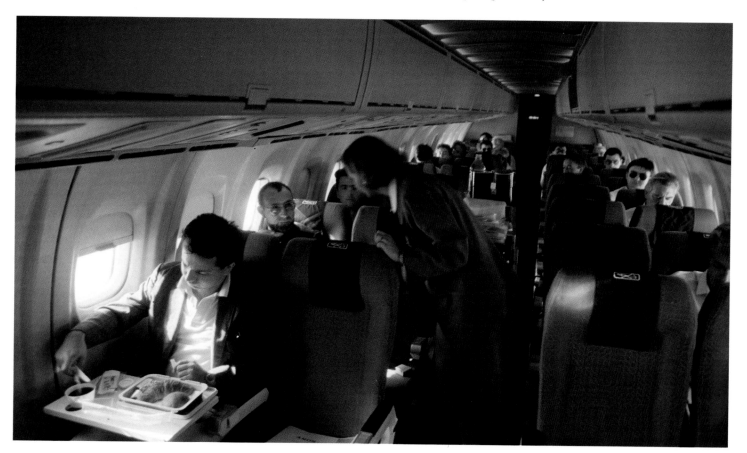

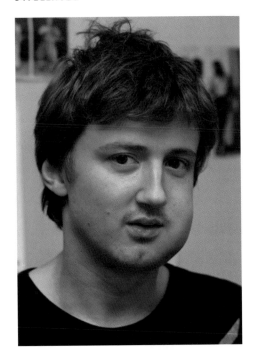

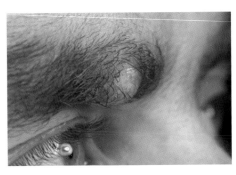

▲ *A sebaceous cyst sometimes appears as a swelling in the area of the eyebrow.*

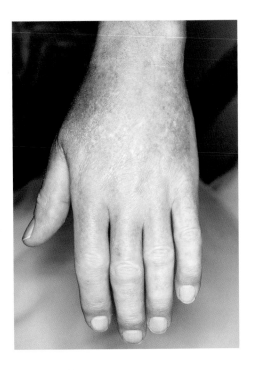

▲ *Wisdom teeth trying to break through can lead to infection. The affected area then becomes swollen in an attempt to fight off the invading bacteria.*

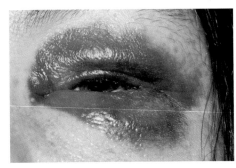

▲ *An injury to the eye causes discoloration and swelling.*

▲ *Scleroderma, an autoimmune disorder, affects the skin and joints of the hand. The joints become swollen and difficult to move and the skin becomes thickened, tight, and shiny.*

size of an orange. They are very common and are not painful. Lumps or cysts in the skin are removed for three reasons: first, to improve the person's appearance and for his or her comfort; second, to make a diagnosis by looking at the tissue under a microscope; third, to remove any lump that is obviously malignant (see Cancer).

## Lymph nodes

The nodes in the neck often swell when a person is suffering from a sore throat or has a fever in a flulike illness. Most of these viral illnesses disappear in two to three days, and the best solution is for the person to go to bed, drink plenty of fluid, and take soluble aspirin or acetaminophen to reduce the temperature and ease headache, sore throat, and general aches and pains.

Sometimes the swollen nodes persist, together with a sore throat, and then infectious mononucleosis may be suspected, especially if the patient is a teenager or a young adult.

In infectious mononucleosis, all the body's lymphatic nodes and the spleen may be enlarged (see Spleen). It may take some time to recover completely from this condition, which often leaves the sufferer feeling lethargic and debilitated.

## Breasts

The breasts should be examined regularly for swellings. They sometimes vary in size and texture during the menstrual cycle and will also enlarge during pregnancy. The best time to examine them is just after a period (see Breasts). If, on examination, a woman does find any lump or swelling, she should always see her doctor. Many breast lumps are not serious, but cancer in a breast should be treated without delay, as the chance of a cure is high if it is diagnosed and treated immediately (see Mammography).

## Abdomen

Swelling of the abdomen has many causes. Constipation caused by too little fiber in the diet is common. Many women find that their abdomen distends before a period and returns to normal afterward. This is caused by hormonal changes.

Painful sudden swelling of the abdomen may be due to intestinal obstruction or another acute cause, and medical attention should be sought. Abdominal swelling without any pain may also be caused by the enlargement of one or more of the organs within the abdomen, or by fluid, and should be reported to a doctor immediately.

## Ruptures

A hernia, or rupture, is a swelling containing intestine that has pressed through a weak point of the muscular wall of the abdomen so that a loop of intestine lies just under the skin. In babies and young children the most common hernias are an umbilical hernia at the navel and an inguinal hernia in the groin. An inguinal hernia is a lump in the groin that enlarges or appears on coughing, and may pass into the scrotum in males. Umbilical hernias normally disappear spontaneously by the age of five. Inguinal hernias can appear at any age and usually need surgery because of the risk of trapping the intestine and causing obstruction and gangrene. If a hernia is large, the intestine is unlikely to get trapped and a truss may be the best treatment. It is a device that presses on the weakness in the muscular abdominal wall to prevent the intestine from emerging (see Hernia).

*See also:* **Glands; Heart disease; Infection and infectious diseases; Infectious mononucleosis; Lumpectomy; Lymphatic system**

# Symptoms

**How does a doctor know when babies are sick? They can't talk about their symptoms.**

Babies show signs of illness like diarrhea and vomiting, but often doctors rely upon the intuition of the mother. Sometimes, there are obvious upsets in a baby's behavior such as crying, not eating, and sleeplessness. At other times, the mother might suspect that the baby is sick even if there is no real evidence. Doctors always try and find out from the mother as much as they can, since a mother is most aware of how her baby is feeling. The doctor will then make a diagnosis from this and from an examination.

**Do all serious illnesses give rise to symptoms?**

No, and this is both a good and a bad thing. On the one hand, it is obviously a good thing that people don't necessarily have to suffer unpleasant symptoms like the horrifying pain caused by blockage in one of the coronary arteries (main blood vessels to the heart). On the other hand, some diseases that might be treatable in their early stages can go unnoticed until it is too late. So symptoms can be both unpleasant and a valuable early warning at the same time.

**I get a severe pain in my teeth, yet my dentist says the trouble is in my sinuses. Why is this?**

Many different conditions and diseases can cause pain at a place away from the center of the trouble. This is called the radiation of pain. Doctors can gain useful information by finding out where pain radiates to. Heart pain, for example, may be felt in the chest but can spread to the arms, shoulders, and jaw. Sometimes, it is felt only in these unconnected places.

---

**To a doctor, symptoms are the primary means of discovering what is wrong with a patient. To a patient suffering, symptoms are what prompt him or her to seek help from a doctor.**

Unpleasant or persistent symptoms are usually what impel a person to consult a doctor in the hope of having them relieved. The symptom being complained about is often just one of the clues a doctor has to make a diagnosis. He or she will then treat a patient on the basis of the diagnosis.

## What are symptoms?

Many people get confused about what symptoms really are. In effect, a symptom is any change in the body or its functions that intrudes sufficiently upon a person's awareness to cause him or her to associate it with a possible illness. These physical or mental sensations can range all the way from a pain in the stomach after eating, to amnesia after an accident. The range of symptoms is enormous, and people suffering from the same underlying illness can experience and describe the way they feel in vastly different ways. This can makes it difficult for a doctor to interpret, from the patients' own words, what they are actually experiencing, but a description of a patient's symptoms is a doctor's primary means of diagnosis, whereby he or she can establish what direction to pursue in tracking down the nature of the patient's illness. When the doctor takes what is called a history—asking diverse questions about the patient's life and general health—other symptoms often come to light. These are often complaints that the patient thought were unconnected with whatever he or she was suffering from. For instance,

**REFERRED PAIN**

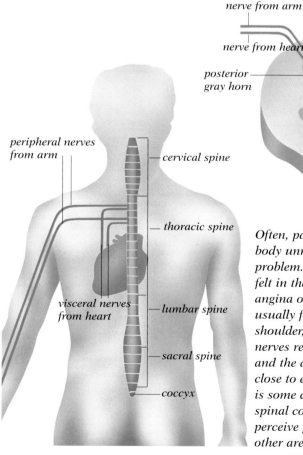

*Often, pain can be felt in an area of the body unrelated to the site of the actual problem. For instance, as well as the pain felt in the center of the chest caused by angina or even a heart attack, victims usually feel pain in the left arm, the left shoulder, and even the jaw. Because nerves relaying pain from both the heart and the arm enter the spinal cord quite close to each other, it is thought that there is some crossover of nerve signals in the spinal cord that causes the brain to perceive pain in the arm as well as in other areas of the body.*

## Some common symptoms and what they mean

| SYMPTOM | CAUSES | TREATMENT AND DANGERS |
|---|---|---|
| **General and psychiatric** | | |
| Tiredness and weakness | Anemia | Determine the cause of the anemia and treat. Iron deficiency is treated with iron. Untreated anemia can be fatal. |
| | Depression: the most common cause of this complaint | Sometimes this diagnosis is quite clear, with unhappiness and sleep disturbance. At other times physical symptoms appear. Suicide is a risk. |
| | Convalescence | Tiredness and weakness are to be expected after any serious illness. It takes a long time to get over a simple viral infection. |
| | Uremia (raised level of breakdown products in the blood, particularly urea): indicates failure of the kidneys | The work of the kidneys has to be taken over by dialysis—using a kidney machine—or transplantation. Without treatment kidney failure can prove fatal. |
| | Addison's disease (lack of steroid hormone) | Replacement of the steroid hormones. The disease is easy to diagnose once suspected. |
| Hallucinations (hearing voices) | Schizophrenia | There are many symptoms of schizophrenia, but hearing voices and paranoia are among the most common. Treatment with drugs controls these symptoms in most cases. |
| | Toxic confusional state | Symptoms of confusion, plus additional features like hallucinations, can occur in any serious illness, particularly in the elderly, and people with a high fever. |
| Anxiety | As well as being a symptom this is a disease in its own right. | Treatment is by many different means, including behavior therapy, psychotherapy, and drugs. Long-lasting anxiety can be very difficult to conquer, despite all the different sorts of treatment available. |
| | Thyrotoxicosis (overactive thyroid gland) | Can be almost indistinguishable from pure anxiety, but blood tests make the diagnosis. Treatment is by pills, surgery, or a radioactive iodine drink. |
| Fever | Usually caused by any sort of infection, but can be caused by tumors or dead tissue | An attempt to identify the organism causing the infection is made, and antibiotic drugs are used if they are effective against the organism concerned. |
| **Head and nervous system** | | |
| Headache | Migraine | In migraine the headache is usually on just one side of the head. |
| | Tension headache: headache without obvious cause | This is a common condition and affect up to 20 percent of people. Most episodes are not serious and subside with painkillers and rest. |
| | Brain tumor | Although there is no denying that brain tumors can cause headaches, it is very uncommon for them to cause headache with no other problem, and they can contribute to only a minute fraction of headaches. |
| | Sinusitis: the ache is more in the face and the teeth, along cheeks | Quitting smoking is essential. Antibiotics and decongestants help. |
| | Temporal arteritis: pain and irritation in the head and scalp | This odd disease is caused by inflammation of the arteries and responds dramatically to treatment with steroids. If untreated, blindness can result. |
| Weakness, complete or partial paralysis | Trauma or diseases that destroy nerves from the brain, through the spinal cord, down to individual nerves or muscles. Common causes are strokes and multiple sclerosis. | There is little in the way of curative treatment, but much can be done with physical therapy to reeducate and rehabilitate the parts of the body that are unaffected. |

## Some common symptoms and what they mean

| SYMPTOM | CAUSES | TREATMENT AND DANGERS |
|---|---|---|
| **Lungs, heart, and chest** | | |
| Chest pain | Angina or a heart attack, depending on duration and severity. Typically, the pain feels crushing and is in the center of the chest, often spreading to the arms and neck. | Pills reduce the severity and frequency of angina attacks, and surgery may be performed to provide an improved blood supply to the heart. The treatment of a heart attack is to give aspirin or a clot-dispersing drug and monitor in a hospital. |
| | Pleurisy: a pain felt anywhere in the chest on breathing | May be a complication of pneumonia, in which case antibiotics are appropriate; or it may just occur on its own accord, in which case painkillers are used. |
| Breathlessness | Heart failure: the heart fails to pump adequately, so fluid collects in the tissues | ACE inhibitor drugs to improve blood supply to heart, kidneys, and brain. Diuretics to clear tissue fluid. Although heart failure can be very serious, patients can have a minor degree of heart failure for years. |
| | Acute bronchitis: with a cough and pneumonia | Infection in the chest both blocks off the bronchial tubes and causes inflammation of the lung tissue. Antibiotics are the usual treatment. |
| | Chronic bronchitis with or without emphysema | A long-term disease causing breathlessness by inflammation of the tubes with excessive phlegm production (chronic bronchitis), or destruction of lung tissue (emphysema). No curative treatment in most cases. Usually caused by smoking. |
| | Asthma: coughing and wheezing | There are now many effective drugs that reduce the frequency, duration, and severity of attacks. |
| Hemoptysis: coughing up of blood | Cancer of the lung, tuberculosis, bronchitis, and bronchiectasis (destruction of bronchi walls) | Because there are serious causes it is essential to see your doctor and have this sign investigated. |

someone who goes to the doctor complaining of weight loss might be asked whether he or she likes hot or cold weather. This might seem irrelevant to the patient, but weight loss and intolerance of heat are clear symptoms of an overactive thyroid gland (see Thyroid). When examining a patient, a doctor looks for signs. These are objective observations, whereas a patient's symptoms are necessarily subjective.

The timing of symptoms is important in forming a diagnosis, and patients have to try and remember when any symptom that is being complained of first occurred, how long it lasted, and how often it happened. As well as knowing the timing of symptoms, the doctor will want to know what, if anything, brings the symptoms on. Sometimes food, or certain types of food, can bring on a burning

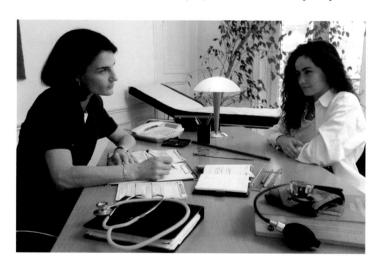

▲ *To arrive at a diagnosis, a doctor asks a patient many questions about lifestyle and symptoms.*

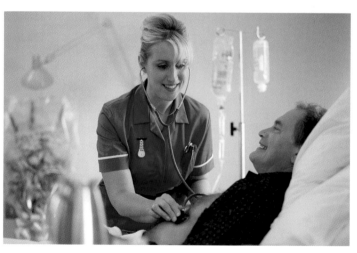

▲ *A physical examination is a necessary element in the process of checking a patient's symptoms.*

## Some common symptoms and what they mean

| SYMPTOM | CAUSES | TREATMENT AND DANGERS |
|---|---|---|
| **Abdomen and gastrointestinal system** | | |
| Dyspepsia: upper abdominal pain | Gastric and duodenal ulceration | Treatment is to reduce the effect of stomach acid which causes the ulcers. Alternatively, the production of acid can be stopped by drugs or surgery. Ulcers can bleed internally and emergency surgery may be needed. |
| | Cholecystitis: gallstones | Removal of the gallbladder |
| | Esophagitis and hiatus hernia | Treatment with drugs |
| Acute abdominal pain, severe pain of sudden origin with a hard, tender abdomen | Many causes: especially anything that inflames the peritoneum (membrane lining the inside of the abdomen), such as appendicitis or spillage of intestinal contents through a perforation (burst ulcer) | This is known as an acute abdomen and the treatment of such problems commonly involves emergency surgery. If you develop an acute abdominal pain, seek medical help as early as possible. |
| Constipation | Many causes | A high-fiber diet is the best treatment, with laxatives needed only rarely. |
| Diarrhea | Gastroenteritis: associated with vomiting | The infection will settle spontaneously. Keep taking as much fluid as possible. |
| | Colitis, when there is also blood and mucus in the feces | Ulcerative colitis is a common type of colitis which usually responds well to drug treatment. The similar Crohn's disease produces colitis as well. |
| **Appetite and weight** | | |
| Thirst | Diabetes, when there is also weight loss, and copious urine is passed | Insulin in the younger diabetic; pills alone may be sufficient for many older diabetics. The urine should always be tested for sugar in anyone (even a baby) who is losing weight, has excessive thirst, and is passing a large volume of urine. |
| Obesity | Constitutional: related to an excess food intake for that particular person | The only treatment is dieting, which may be combined with an exercise program. Dangers: probably an increased risk of heart attack in younger people, and an increased risk of diabetes. |
| | Cushing's syndrome: overactive adrenal glands causing obesity (with other symptoms) | This is a rare disease that is easy to recognize and accounts for many people's thinking they can blame obesity on glands. |
| Loss of appetite and weight loss | Many causes, including most of the serious diseases such as cancer | It is rare for a cancer to show up as weight loss with no other symptoms or signs. Isolated weight loss is often found to be caused by mild depression. |

pain in the upper abdomen. Milk or antacid pills may alleviate the pain, and this makes diagnosis of indigestion virtually certain.

### Treatment of symptoms

It is very important that a diagnosis is made before treatment is given. For example, if a pain was treated before diagnosis and it was due to a condition that became progressively worse or needed urgent treatment, the patient, although not in pain, could die. If someone with severe pain in the abdomen were given a shot of morphine, the doctor would not have any idea about what might be going on. If the pain were due to an inflamed appendix, the patient could be pain-free but the condition could worsen until the appendix ruptured (see Appendicitis). If surgery were not performed, the patient could die.

There are some symptoms that it is safe to treat, even when the doctor is not sure what is wrong. It is safe to take an aspirin for a minor headache. Other times, treatment is given to relieve a particular symptom even though the medicine has no effect on the cause of the trouble. This is symptomatic treatment. The use of simple painkillers or cough medicines is a good example. One of the main skills involved in a doctor's job is to know when this kind of simple treatment is safe and appropriate.

*See also:* **Diagnosis; Indigestion**

# Syphilis

## Questions and Answers

**Why do people regard syphilis with so much fear?**

For three main reasons. First, because unless treated it is capable of causing serious brain and arterial damage; it may lead to death in 5 to 10 percent of untreated patients, or to permanent disability. Second, because it is very difficult to identify in the early stages except by a doctor. Third, because if it does escape detection the patient has what is virtually a life sentence of uncertainty and worry about if, when, and where the condition may strike, since it is able to affect almost all the systems in the body, especially the brain and the largest artery (aorta).

**Is syphilis difficult to diagnose?**

No. There are reliable blood tests that can make the diagnosis in a matter of hours, regardless of the stage of the disease. However, unless a doctor is consulted and made aware—by the history or clinical features—of the possibility, these tests will never be made and the patient may progress to the dangerous later stages.

In its early stages, syphilis can be very difficult for patients to recognize. This difficulty in detection is due to several different factors. First, the sore that characterizes early syphilis often takes a long time to develop, sometimes as long as three months, so that people are likely not to associate it with the event that caused it. In many cases, possibly as many as one-third, no sore occurs and the first stage is silent. Another problem is that the sore or ulcer is painless and, furthermore, it heals by itself, without any treatment, in the course of a few days. It is therefore understandable that all these factors tend to make the patient think that he or she doesn't have anything very serious, and consequently no medical advice is sought about the situation.

**Of all the sexually transmitted diseases, syphilis is, after AIDS, the most dangerous; if undetected, it may eventually cause disablement or death. People should therefore seek immediate medical attention if the disease is suspected.**

Syphilis is not the most common sexually transmitted disease (STD), but it is potentially one of the most serious if it is not treated within the first few years. If it remains undiagnosed it continues—like a life sentence—through three progressively more serious stages. However, in a proportion of untreated patients it seems to clear up spontaneously; the reason for this is still unknown.

In the primary and secondary stages, syphilis is an infectious disease of the sex organs and sometimes of the skin and lining of the mouth. It later passes into a dormant, or latent, stage, when no signs of the disease can be seen and the patient has no symptoms of illness. This stage may last from five to as many as 50 years, and it is only after all that time that some of those infected enter into the third stage. In these people, syphilis is often a chronic, crippling, and, for some, a killing disease. Indeed, in the United States alone, hundreds die from it every year.

## Progress of the disease

The syphilis germ, shaped like a tiny corkscrew, called *Treponema pallidum*, is a spirochete. About a thousand of these may be acquired during intercourse with an infected person (see Intercourse). Every 30 hours or so each germ grows and divides into two, each two into four, each four into eight, and so on. When the first sign of the disease appears, many millions of germs are already present in the victim's body.

**The first stage:** In the first or primary stage, the disease usually shows itself by the appearance of an ulcer or sore on or in the sex organs (see Sores). This ulcer is completely painless and is often neglected for this reason. Occasionally, the primary sore may appear on other parts of the

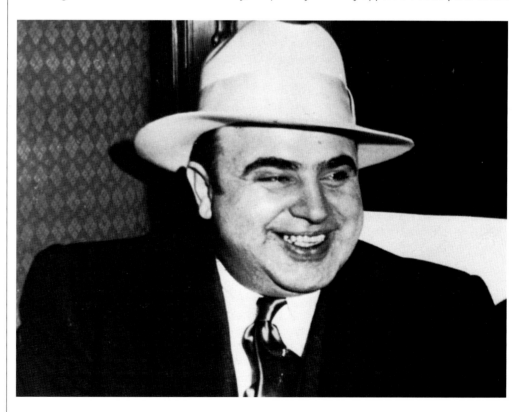

▲ *The notorious Chicago gangster Al Capone is still smiling as he is escorted to begin an 11-year prison sentence. Capone had syphilis, from which he later died.*

**Can syphilis be diagnosed just by doing a blood test?**

Yes. The standard test for syphilis is called the VDRL (venereal disease research laboratory) test. It is used worldwide and is cheap and simple. It is used to diagnose, to test for the effectiveness of treatment, and to test for reinfection after successful treatment. In active infection, the test remains positive with progressive dilution of the blood sample. The VDRL test becomes positive during the primary stage of syphilis, and during the secondary stage it will remain positive even at a dilution of 32 times. Effective treatment can be demonstrated by a sharp drop in the dilution capable of giving a positive result. Syphilis can also be diagnosed early by microscopic examination of the fluid from the base of the primary sore (chancre). This shows the characteristic spiral-shaped bacteria called spirochetes.

**I have read about something called latent syphilis. What exactly is this?**

This is the stage in which the disease is inactive. It follows the secondary stage, in which the disease is often virulent, and may lead to the last stage, when the really unpleasant consequences of syphilis occur. In the dormant, or latent, stage, the patient has no indication of illness, and the only evidence that he or she has the disease will be the discovery, usually at a prenatal examination or when the patient donates blood, that the blood tests are positive; or when blood tests are performed because of suspected contact with the infection.

There is little risk of passing the disease on to anybody else through sexual intercourse during the latent stage, but women can unwittingly pass the condition on to the fetus if they become pregnant.

This is why all pregnant women are tested for syphilis. Should the test turn out to be positive, it is possible to give the pregnant woman treatment which, if given early enough, will prevent the baby from being born with syphilis.

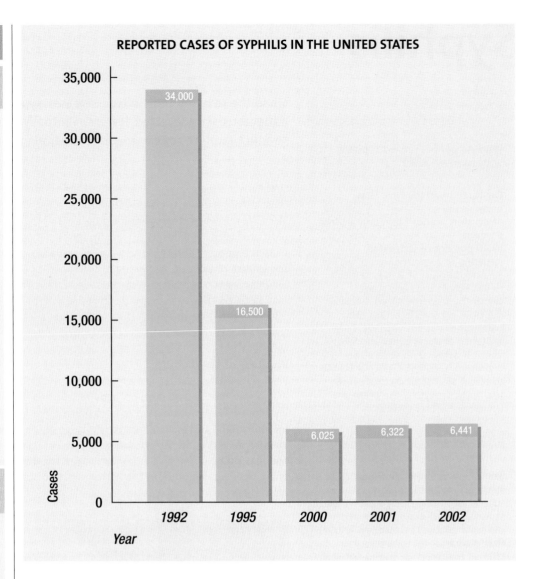

### REPORTED CASES OF SYPHILIS IN THE UNITED STATES

Cases (vertical axis): 0, 5,000, 10,000, 15,000, 20,000, 25,000, 30,000, 35,000

Year (horizontal axis):
- 1992: 34,000
- 1995: 16,500
- 2000: 6,025
- 2001: 6,322
- 2002: 6,441

body, for example, in or around the mouth or on the fingers. In homosexual men, the sore may appear on or at the opening of the anus. Primary sores (there may be several) appear about 21 days after the infecting intercourse, but this incubation period may be as short as 9 days or, rarely, as long as 90 days. In some patients there is nothing to be seen; in a few, the sore may be only a small crack in the skin.

A week or two after the sore appears, painless lumps (enlarged glands) can be found in the groin (see Glands). These swellings show that the body's defenses are working to try to kill off the invading germs (see Swellings). In some women with syphilis, the primary ulcer or sore is internal, and therefore may pass unnoticed. After days or weeks the ulcer, even if untreated, heals. This gives those who have not been treated the impression that all is well, but this is not so. If the disease is not treated the germs may invade almost any organ of the body, something that occurs in about 40 percent of patients.

**The second stage:** This stage shows itself as a generalized rash. This rash is not itchy and may appear anywhere on the body. It can be so slight and faint that it is often ignored. There may also be sores in the mouth or in the throat, or around the sex organs. Headache, fever, and aches in the bones may occur, and there is often enlargement of the glands in the neck and elsewhere. These symptoms of secondary syphilis come and go if the disease is not treated.

**The dormant, or latent, stage:** If the infection is not diagnosed, or not treated properly, the rash and other symptoms wax and wane and eventually disappear. The disease then enters the dormant, or latent, stage: this can last from five to 50 years and will be wholly symptom-free. The disease is no longer so infectious, but women who have undetected syphilis can pass on the condition to their fetus if they become pregnant even several years later (see Fetus; Pregnancy). This may result in a baby's being born dead, deformed, or diseased.

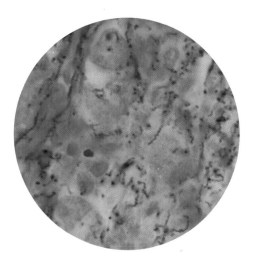

▲ *The cause of syphilis is the* Treponema pallidum *spirochete.*

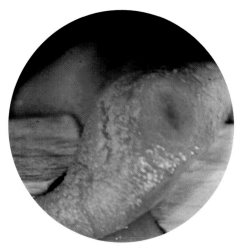

▲ *In the primary stage, the tongue becomes ulcerated.*

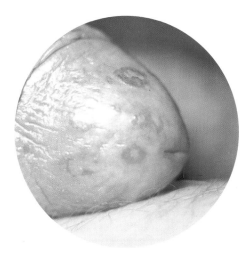

▲ *In the secondary stage, a rash and sores appear on the sex organs.*

**The third stage:** About a third of those who have undetected syphilis suffer sooner or later from skin ulcers, syphilitic heart disease, syphilitic paralysis, insanity, blindness, or deafness. In this stage so much damage has often been done by the germs over many years that treatment can only halt the progress of the disease; but in some the mechanical damage progresses, even though the infection can be cleared. In the earlier stages, syphilis can be cured completely and permanently.

## Detection and treatment

In the primary and secondary stages of syphilis the disease can be diagnosed by scraping the primary sore or one of the parts of the rash, taking some of the fluid which then oozes out, and finding the tiny corkscrew bacterium in it under the microscope. Six weeks after infection, substances that show the body's defenses are working can be detected by a blood test, but before that time the blood test will be negative. In the latent stage, only a blood test will detect syphilis. This test is given to all people attending a genitourinary clinic (see Screening).

All pregnant women attending prenatal clinics have a blood test for syphilis as a matter of course. If the disease is detected, they are treated immediately and usually go on to have perfectly healthy children. Every donation of blood for transfusion is, by law, tested for syphilis before it can be given to another person. Blood tests are also done selectively for patients who are under investigation in the hospital because syphilis may actually imitate other illnesses.

At all stages penicillin is the chosen treatment (see Penicillin). It is given as a course of daily injections; the patient attends after working hours if possible. Then every treated person is asked to attend for two years at monthly, and later three-monthly, intervals for an examination and a blood test.

Only in this way can the doctor guarantee that the cure is permanent. Treatment given in the first year of the latent stage is curative, but after that all that may be done is to halt the progress of the disease. It is thought that some cases of unsuspected syphilis may have been cured by incidental penicillin given for other infections.

## Warning

Syphilis is a great cheater. It is curable, but only if it is recognized and correctly diagnosed early on. The problem is that it is often extremely difficult to detect at this stage. The symptoms may sometimes take three months to develop and the victim may not associate a sore developing in March with a casual sexual encounter at Christmas. Probably as many as a third of all people who develop syphilis fail to detect the sore and can pass through the primary stage with nothing to show, and thus be completely unaware that they have the disease.

A number never produce a proper sore, but only a rather insignificant crack in the skin, which may be difficult to find and may require a doctor to diagnose. Also, the sore is painless, and patients tend not to go to a doctor with things that do not hurt them; moreover, the sore goes away by itself, even if no treatment is given.

So any person who thinks that there is even the slightest chance that he or she may have been with somebody who has syphilis should go to a genitourinary clinic and find out for sure; the disease is much too dangerous and insidious for a person to be in any doubt about it. Clinics exist in most cities throughout the United States, and a person can usually go without having to make an appointment.

▼ *This is a graphic representation of the sort of symptoms that are associated with the secondary stage of syphilis.*

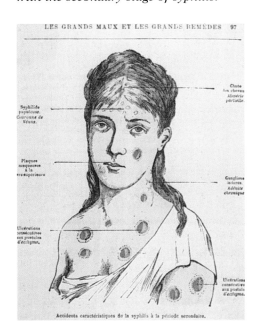

*See also:* **Bacteria; Blood donor; Deafness; Prenatal care; Rashes; Sexually transmitted diseases; Ulcers**

# Syringing

**My ears seem to make a lot of wax. Will they need syringing regularly to clear out the wax?**

Wax is a natural substance secreted into the ear canal and it acts as a cleanser. It picks up dust from the canal and passes out toward the edge of the ear. You can then wipe it away without poking anything into the canal. Your ears certainly do not need syringing unless the wax hardens and builds up in the canal, causing irritation, infection, or deafness.

**My four-year-old son had a runny ear, which I thought was due to excess wax, but the doctor gave him antibiotics. Why was this?**

You certainly did the right thing in taking your son to have his ears checked. Sometimes a runny ear is due to wax, but often it is caused when an infection in the middle ear breaks through the eardrum, causing a hole or perforation in the drum to let the pus leak out. This may be apparently painless, or the ear may be painful until the drum is perforated, when the ache caused by the pressure is released. It is better that a runny ear is due simply to wax and not to perforation, which can lead to deafness unless treated quickly. The perforation itself causes some deafness, which disappears when the hole in the drum heals.

**Why did my doctor ask if I felt dizzy when I had my ear syringed?**

If the water is squirted too forcibly on the eardrum, you may feel dizzy because the inner ear structures that help in balancing are affected. These lie near the drum and are affected if the water used is too warm or too cold. Sometimes a patient may react so strongly to a high or low water temperature that he or she may lose balance and fall down.

**Deafness and irritation could indicate that your ears need syringing. A doctor can soon remove the cause of the problem—hard earwax—by gently squirting water into the ears.**

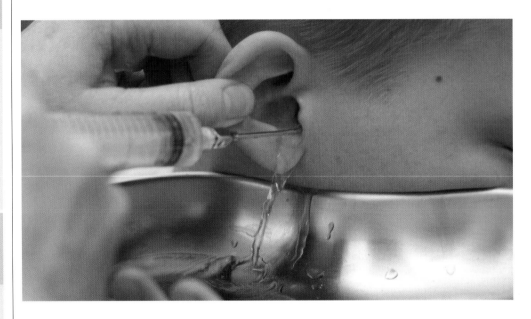

▲ *A doctor squirts warm water into the ear to remove wax deposits.*

Usually ears are syringed to rid the outer canal of wax, which may build up and harden and result in impaired hearing. The basic process involves squirting water gently into the ear to soften the wax and to help dislodge it (see Earwax).

## Conditions requiring syringing

Wax, or cerumen, is the normal secretion of the ceruminous glands that are found in the outer part of the external ear canal. Mixed with the wax is keratin, a horny material from the surface of the skin that is normally rubbed off in tiny quantities; and sebum, the greasy lubricant of the skin. Dust and other materials also find their way into the external ear passage, especially in people who have occupations such as coal mining. The amount and texture of the wax secreted vary considerably. Most people form a small amount of soft wax that works its way, unnoticed, out of the ears. It is likely to be produced in large amounts, and to become harder, only in the middle and later years of life.

Children are rarely affected by hard wax, but they sometimes put things into their ears, such as beads, pips, seeds, and small stones. In this case, nothing should be poked into the ear to try to remove the object, since poking is likely to cause rupture of the eardrum. Cotton-covered sticks are dangerous; they will push the object in farther. Instead, a doctor should be consulted. He or she will try to flush the object out with water using a syringe, while looking frequently into the ear. Or he or she might use a small hook or probe and look through an auriscope (an instrument for examining ears). If a young child is involved, or if the object is deeply embedded, general anesthesia will be necessary. Insects also sometimes get into the ear, particularly small flies; these can cause irritation. The best treatment is to drop warm olive oil into the ear; this can be done safely at home. This kills the fly so a doctor can easily syringe it out later.

## Wax buildup

When hard wax fills the ear canal it causes deafness (see Deafness). In an elderly person whose hearing is already poor, or in anyone who has diminished hearing, excess wax may make a huge

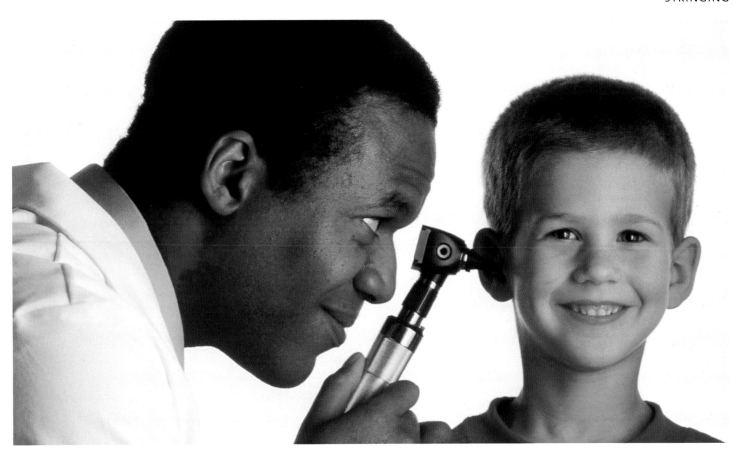

difference. The wax may cause irritation or may cause noises in the ear by pressing on the eardrum, and, occasionally, balance will be affected, causing feelings of unsteadiness (see Hearing).

## Procedure

After a doctor has prescribed syringing, a patient will be told to use a few drops of warm olive or almond oil in the ear once or twice a day for seven to fourteen days in order to soften the wax before treatment. The instrument used for the treatment is usually a large

▲ *A doctor uses an auriscope to inspect for wax buildup in the outer ear.*

metal syringe with a rounded nozzle, although some operators prefer a rubber syringe. The patient is protected with towels and plastic sheeting, and is usually asked to hold a kidney-shaped dish beneath the ear to catch the water and any pieces of wax. The fluid used is usually warm water, but sodium bicarbonate or saline solutions may be used. The temperature of the water is important: it should be no hotter or colder than body temperature, 98.6°F (37°C). The external ear is drawn upward and back in order to straighten the ear canal. The syringe nozzle is kept away from the eardrum and the water is directed at the sides and ceiling of the ear canal; there should be no pain during this process. If any wax remains, the patient is sent away with further advice to soften it with oil, and the syringing is then repeated a week later. Excess fluid should be mopped up from the ear canal; stagnant fluid may result in an infection (otitis externa).

## Dangers and outlook

Damaging an eardrum is the main danger. If a perforation should result, then infection can enter the middle ear, resulting in deafness, and may spread to the spongy bone behind the ear (mastoid process). Syringing while there is a perforation can spread infection and force bacteria into the blood vessels and bone; antibiotics may be needed. The skin of the external ear canal can get damaged and bleed, or become infected. It usually heals quickly; healing can be helped with antibiotic and steroid drops.

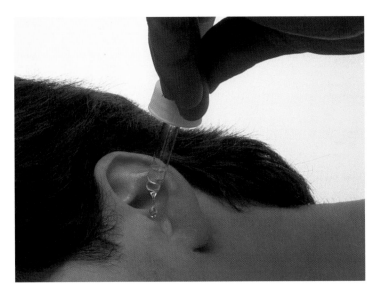

▲ *Prior to syringing, the doctor will tell you to drop oil into your ear for a week or so to soften the wax.*

See also: **Bacteria; Otitis**

# INDEX

Headings and page numbers in **bold** refer to complete articles. Page numbers in *italics* refer to illustrations or their captions.

## A

abdomen
  pain 2152
  swelling 2148
abortion, sterilization not recommended at the same time 2068
abruption, placental 2081
abscess, meibomian 2113
acetaminophen (Tylenol; Tempra), overdose 2093
acute abdomen 2152
adaptation syndrome 2099
Addison's disease 2072, 2150
adhesions, stiffness and 2077
adrenaline (epinephrine) 2064, 2085, 2099
allergies 2145, 2147
altitudes, high, training at 2052
aminophylline 2085
amniocentesis, spina bifida and 2038
amphetamines 2083, 2084
amylase (ptyalin) 2063, *2064*
anemia, hemolytic 2045
anesthesiologists *2137*
anesthetics *2041*, 2134, 2135
aneurysms, berry 2107
angina 2067, *2149*, 2151
ankles
  edema 2146
  sprained *2057*, 2145
  stiffness 2079
antidepressants 2084
antiseptics 2135, *2137*
anxiety 2150
aphasia 2030
apnea, in babies 2117
arms
  broken *2048*, *2049*
  stiffness 2078
arteries, hardening 2121
arteriovenous anomaly 2108
arteritis, temporal 2073, 2150
arthritis
  stiffness and 2077–2078
  treatment 2049, 2072–2073
artificial insemination 2141
aseptic techniques 2135–2136
aspirin 2079, 2111
assertiveness training 2104
asthma 2050, 2072
atherosclerosis, strokes and 2107

## B

babies
  illness diagnosed in 2149
  sudden infant death syndrome (SIDS) 2116–2117
back, stiff 2076, 2078
barium liquids, enemas 2096

biopsy 2025–2026
birth
  pain relief *2041*
  umbilical cord accidents 2094
bites and stings *2145*, 2147
blood
  sugar 2121
  tests *2024–2025*
blood pressure, measurement *2036*
bowel
  intussusception 2095–2096
  obstruction 2094
braces 2048
  dental 2050
brain, speech and 2029
brain damage and disease
  embolisms 2107–2108
  hemorrhage 2108, *2109*
  herniation 2096
  thrombosis in the arteries 2107
  tumors 2150
brain surgery *2134*
breasts, examination 2148
breathlessness 2151
bronchitis 2151

## C

caffeine *2083–2085*
carbohydrates, dietary 2063–2064, 2120, 2121
carbolic acid 2135
cartilage, torn 2055
casts, plaster *2048*
cerebral palsy 2022
cervix, Pap smear 2071
chest, pains 2151
child development, speech *2028*, 2030–2031
children
  speech problems 2028, 2030, 2032, *2033*, 2058–2061
  sunburn 2128, 2129
chlorpromazine 2126
cholecystitis 2152
chyme 2088
cleft palate, speech and 2030
coffee *2083*, 2084
cognitive reappraisal 2104
colitis 2152
colon
  cancer 2022
  spastic 2022–2023
compresses 2056, 2113
conception *2035*
constipation, treatment *2132*, 2133, 2152
Cushing's syndrome 2152
cyclic AMP 2085
cyst
  eyelid (meibomian cyst) 2112
  sebaceous *2147*, *2148*

## D

dandruff, sties and 2112
deafness, earwax and 2156–2157
depression, and suicide *2123*, 2124
dermatitis, seborrheic 2112, 2113

desferrioxamine 2093
diabetes 2082, 2120, 2121
diarrhea 2152
digoxin 2083
disaccharides 2120, *2121*
dislocation 2055
  hip 2048
doxapram *2085*
dreaming 2114
drug abuse, amphetamines 2084
drugs
  photosensitizing 2126
  taken as suppositories *2132–2133*
dysarthria 2031, 2033
dyslexia 2028
dyspepsia 2152

## E

eardrums, perforated 2156, 2157
ears, syringing 2156–2157
edema
  angioneurotic 2145, 2147
  nephrotic 2146
ejaculation 2035
elbow, stiffness 2078
emetics 2092–2093
enemas, barium 2096
epidural injections *2041*
epinephrine *see* adrenaline
euthanasia 2125
exercise
  menstrual cycle and 2052
  stitch following *2086*, 2087
  for stroke patients *2111*
  warm-ups before *2055*, 2086
eyes, foreign bodies in 2047

## F

face, puffiness on waking 2146
fallopian tubes, sterilization involving 2069, *2070*, 2071
feces, samples 2025
feet
  stiffness 2079
  swollen on air journeys 2145, *2147*
fevers 2150
fingers
  splints *2049*
  stiffness 2078
fishhooks, embedded in the skin 2047
folic acid 2037, 2039
food poisoning 2062
fractures
  hairline 2048
  splinting *2048*, *2049*
  sports 2050–2051, 2054
fructose *2121*

## G

gallbladder, removal 2134
gastritis *2088*, 2089, 2090
gastroenteritis 2089, 2151, 2152
glandular fever *see* infectious mononucleosis

glomerulonephritis 2097
glucagon *2064*
glucose 2120, 2121
  stored as glycogen *2064*, 2120
glycogen *2064*, 2120

## H

hallucinations 2150
hallux rigidus 2079
headache 2150
head injuries, brain herniation and 2096
heart
  murmurs 2074
  pain 2149
  strangulation of 2096
  valves 2067, *2136*
heart attack 2024, 2108, *2149*, 2151
heart failure 2083, 2146, 2151
Heimlich maneuver *2119*
hematoma 2096
hemoptysis 2151
hemorrhoids 2095, *2096*
hernia 2094, 2095, *2095*, 2096, 2148
histopathology 2026
human chorionic gonadotropin (HCG) 2024
hydrocortisone 2078, 2079, 2133
hypertension (high blood pressure), and stroke 2107, 2111
hypoglycemia 2121
hysterectomy 2069, 2071

## I

ice therapy *2051*
incontinence, spinal cord damage and 2040
indigestion, persistent 2090
infectious mononucleosis (glandular fever) 2044, 2046, 2148
infertility, sperm and 2034, 2035
insulin *2064*, 2121
internal examination 2027
intestines
  intussusception 2095–2096
  peristalsis 2023
  strangulation 2094–*2095*
  tumor removal 2136
iron pills, overdose 2093
irritable bowel syndrome (IBS) 2022

## J

joints
  injections into 2078
  sports injuries 2054–2055
  stiffness 2076, 2077–2079

## K

kala-azar *2046*
keratoses, solar 2127
knee
  stiffness 2079
  torn cartilage 2055

## L

lactic acid 2076
lactose, intolerance 2023
laparoscopy *2138*
larynx, stenosis 2067
legs
    fractures 2048, *2049*
    stiffness 2079
leukemia, enlarged spleen 2046
ligaments, sprained 2056–2057
ligatures 2137
light, effect on the skin 2127
lignocaine 2078
limbs, stiff 2076
lipomas 2147–2148
lisping 2060
liver, glycogen storage *2064*, 2120
liver diseases, the spleen and 2046
living wills 2125
lymph nodes, swollen 2145, 2148

## M

marrow, stem cells 2065
massage 2056, 2078, *2079*
meditation *2104*
melanin 2127
meningocele 2037, *2039*
meningomyelocele *2039*
menstruation, exercise during 2052
methyldopa 2045
microsurgery 2139
migraine 2150
miscarriage 2034
monosaccharides 2120, *2121*
MRSA (methicillin-resistant *Staphylococcus aureus*) 2062
multiple sclerosis (MS) 2033, 2040, 2043
muscles
    intercostal 2087
    pulled or strained *2051*, 2054
myelitis 2040, 2043

## N

narcolepsy 2083
nasogastric tubes 2134
neck
    broken 2040
    stiff 2078, *2079*
nerves, spinal *2042*
novocaine 2078

## O

osteoarthritis 2077–2078
ovaries, sterilization involving the 2069, 2071
overdoses
    suicide and 2124
    *see also* stomach pump
oxytetracycline 2126

## P

pain, referred *2149*
Pap smear (cervical smear), after sterilization 2071

paralysis 2150
paraplegia 2043
Parkinson's disease, and speech 2032
peristalsis 2023
personality, A-type and B-type, stress and 2101
perspiration (sweat) 2130–2131
phlegm (sputum), tests 2025
phonation 2029
photosensitivity 2126, 2129
photosynthesis 2063
physical therapy, for stroke victims *2107*, 2110
Pill, the 2107
placebo effect, tonics and 2083
plants, a source of starch 2063
pleurisy, treatment 2151
polysaccharides 2120, *2121*
post-traumatic stress disorder (PTSD) 2102
poultices, bread and starch 2063
pregnancy
    alcohol taken during 2080
    ectopic 2068, 2069, 2070
    folic acid supplements 2037, 2039
    rhesus (Rh) factor and 2081
    smoking during 2080
    stretch marks 2105, *2105*
    swollen ankles 2146, *2147*
    tests for 2024
prickly heat 2130
psychoneuroimmunology 2102
psychotherapy *2114*, 2115
puberty, stretch marks 2105
purple hearts 2083

## Q

quadriplegia 2043

## R

rashes
    photosensitive 2126
    prickly heat 2130
    syphilis 2154, *2155*
reflexes *2040*, 2041
relaxation 2103, 2104
rhesus (Rh) factor 2081
rheumatic fever 2067, 2097
rheumatoid arthritis 2072–2073, 2077

## S

scalded skin syndrome 2062
scalpels 2137–2138
scars, healing 2136
schizophrenia 2150
scleroderma (systemic sclerosis) 2148
sebaceous glands
    cysts 2147, *2148*
    sties and *2112*
semen 2035
seminal vesicles 2035
shellfish, allergy to 2145
shell shock 2102
shoes, sports 2052
shoulder, stiff 2076, 2078, *2079*

sinuses, radiation of pain from 2149
sinusitis, and headaches 2150
skin
    cancer 2024, 2127–2128
    specimens 2024
    swellings 2147–*2148*
smoking, during pregnancy 2080
**spastic colon 2022–2023**
**specimens 2024–2026**
**speculum 2027**
**speech 2028–2031**
    *see also* stammering and stuttering
**speech therapy 2032–2033,** 2110
**sperm 2034–2035**
sphincter, pyloric 2088
**sphygmomanometer 2036**
**spina bifida 2037–2039,** 2041–2043
**spinal cord 2040–2043**
spinal tap 2042
**spleen 2044–2046**
**splinters 2047**
**splints 2048–2049**
**sports injury 2050–2051,** 2052–2055
**sports medicine 2052–2055**
sprains 2048, 2051, 2055, **2056–2057,** 2145
**stammering and stuttering** 2032, **2058–2061**
**staphylococcus 2062**
**starch 2063–2064,** 2121
**stem cell 2065–2066**
**stenosis 2067**
sterilization (microbial) 2135–2136
**sterilization (reproductive) 2068–2071**
**steroids 2072–2073**
**stethoscope 2074–2075**
**stiffness** 2054, **2076–2079**
**stillbirth 2080–2082**
**stimulants 2083–2085**
**stitch 2086–2087**
stitches see sutures
**stomach 2088–2090**
**stomach pump 2091–2093**
strain 2098
**strangulation 2094–2096**
**streptococcus 2097**
**stress 2098–2102,** 2103
**stress management 2103–2104**
**stretch marks 2105–2106**
stroke 2107–2111
strychnine 2084
**sty 2112–2113**
**subconscious 2114–2115**
sucrose 2121
**sudden infant death syndrome** (SIDS) **2116–2117**
**suffocation 2118–2119**
**sugars 2120–2121**
**suicide 2122–2125**
**sunburn 2126–2129**
sunscreen 2128–2129

**sunstroke** (heatstroke) **2130–2131**
**suppositories 2132–2133**
surgeons 2134, 2139–2140
**surgery 2134–2140**
**surrogacy 2141–2143**
**sutures** (stitches) 2136–2137, 2138, **2144**
**swellings 2145–2148**
**symptoms 2149–2152**
syphilis 2042, **2153–2155**
**syringing 2156–2157**

## T

teeth
    pain 2149
    sugar and 2120, 2121
    wisdom *2148*
temperature, regulation 2130–2131
tendons, sports injuries 2054
testicles, temperature 2035
thirst, symptom of diabetes 2152
throat, strep *2097*
thrombosis
    deep vein 2146
    stroke and 2107
thyroid
    cancer 2096
    overactive 2150
tiredness 2150
toes, stiffness 2079
tongue, swallowing the 2118
tonics 2083, 2084
toxic confusional state 2150
transient ischemic attacks 2109, 2111
tumors, pressing on the spinal cord 2043

## U

ulcers *2088*, 2089–2090, 2102, 2138
ultrasound, during pregnancy *2143*
umbilical cord, accidents 2094
uremia, treatment 2150
urine, tests 2024, 2025, *2026*
urticaria 2147

## V

varicose veins, and swollen ankles 2146–2147
VDRL test 2154
vitamin B, B12, deficiency 2043
volvulus neonatorum 2094
vomiting 2088–2089

## W

weakness 2150
weight
    stretch marks and *2105*, 2106
    unexplained loss of 2152
worms, in the feces 2025
wrinkles 2127
wrist, stiffness 2078